I0458240

No HuMan Can Make an Apple

Isabell Thomas

Copyright © Isabell Thomas 2025

All Rights Reserved

No part of this publication may be reproduced, distributed, or transmitted in any form or by any means, including photocopying, recording, or other electronic or mechanical methods, without the author's prior written permission, except in the case of brief quotations embodied in critical reviews and certain other non-commercial uses permitted by copyright law. For permission requests, please get in touch with the author.

Dedication

I dedicate this book to my sister, Sheila, my sister, Angela, my brother, Graham, and my mother and father, who have all passed away but remain with me in spirit.

Acknowledgments

I give thanks to my family.

I am grateful to all those I have learned from, who have given and shown me love, as well as those who have placed their hell-consciousness upon me; I send them love and forgiveness. I also send love to those I have hurt along the way.

About the Author

Isabell had a wide range of interests, from DIY projects and building fences in her free time to working in admin for the Armed Forces. Her curiosity eventually led her to pursue a career as a psychotherapist, but she soon realised that the title only captured a fraction of her true passion. After earning three degrees, including a master's in Psychological Therapies, she found herself losing the desire to pursue a PhD.

Her journey was shaped by a quote she learned at university: "The normal reaction to an abnormal situation." This was further deepened by the loss of family members and her own health struggles, leaving her with unanswered questions. These experiences propelled her into exploring the complexities of life, leading her to write. Although it was a challenging process, she found it transformative, describing the act of writing her book as if it were writing itself.

Isabell also speaks about mental illness and interventions on YouTube:

https://youtu.be/CMQDqcgZBuU?si=omcJ3y_IycgVfJLx

I know of no man with the intelligence to create an apple.

Therefore, I can only look to our Creator,

The one who made the apple, for truth and healing.

Preface

This book wrote itself. I just became the passenger after the realisation that I know of no man who can make an apple.

The circumstances you experience from birth and what you are taught about the world are primarily lies—lies made up of control and obedience. What or how you are is determined by who you act as.

The "who" you act as is derived from a character you built or the egoic character that developed. This character is shaped by likes, dislikes, wants, don't-wants, prejudices, pain, anger, anxiety, and fear. These are the egoic stories.

We are asleep in these stories, living our lives avoiding and chasing because of the made-up stories we have been introduced to. This egoic thinking has driven a wedge between who we really are and the arrogance of the egoic mind, which constantly tries to tell us who we are.

We cannot find who we are or be told who we are because we discover it through the oneness within ourselves. The oneness within us is a space where egoic thinking cannot enter and does not exist.

My Search for the Truth

"John 8:31–32: To the Jews who had believed him, Jesus said, 'If you hold to my teaching, you are really my disciples. Then you will know the truth, and the truth will set you free.'"

I was born with the word *why* indoctrinated into my system, as many children are. I was often shut down with answers like, "It just is," or, "It's just one of those things." This was my first introduction to the world of ignorance, and it continued.

I could only look to the one who made the apple because there is no human being I know of who can create an apple—or many of the wonderful creations on this planet that the human ego has claimed as *mine*. Even our body is a gift. If only we would all wake up and realise that normalising our thoughts and actions does not mean that they are healthy or natural.

I no longer listen to the news or social media, nor do I blindly believe everything said by those with professional labels. I see that behind all labels lies a human being, no matter who we act as or pretend to be. The impact of our upbringing and brainwashing will inevitably seep through those labels.

We can be conditioned very quickly when we neglect ourselves. For example, when a person is unconsciously trained to use a filler word—such as "like" or "obviously"—in every sentence, they often find it difficult to stop, even when it is pointed out to them.

Isabell Thomas

'When I tell the truth, it is not

For the sake of convincing those who

Do not know it,

But for the sake of defending those that do'

William Blake.

Introduction

Imagine a story being told that you are a superior being—that you are the most intelligent being on the planet. What would you do with that?

All creatures on Earth are creations, and no human can make any of them. However, despite man being created after many of the creatures, he believed a lie about himself that not only led him into despair but also began to destroy the planet and the creatures on it.

A war between good and evil unfolded on Earth. Evil lied and divided man from his spirit, enslaving any creature or human who was different with stories of deceit. Man committed horrific and abhorrent acts to demonstrate his supposed superiority, condemning all he deemed inferior or lower.

The only way man could uphold this false narrative of being superior, civilised, and intelligent was to act out evil. He became a "human-doing," casting aside his spiritual being to destroy what the Creator had made, all in the pursuit of money.

Man has constructed a made-up story that glorifies his imagined superiority and intelligence. He has created labels that do not define who he truly is. He has reshaped the world into something unrecognisable from its original form.

It is beyond comprehension how anyone with a professional title can claim the ability to create something as simple as a toenail from nothing. This raises the question: how can anyone assert that another person is inadequate or flawed when they themselves lack the capacity to create a human being? Such claims reveal an extraordinary level of arrogance rooted in the ego.

Man remains a child to evil, chasing an unattainable sense of being "good enough" within the lie. As a "human-doing," he searches for material things to fill the void, but the thirst remains unending. This thirst cannot be quenched within the false narrative of Hell.

We are constantly reminded that nothing is ever good enough. Our phones, appliances, cars, and clothes are perpetually outdated, replaced by something "better." Even cleaning products are advertised as more brilliant each year.

Hell is characterised by an unending and tormenting thirst that remains perpetually unfulfilled (Luke 16:22–24).

Life in the Conscious State

Dr David Hawkins (2005) articulated the levels of consciousness. He determined that the field from which consciousness arises has always existed, and because it has always been, it will always be. This means that death is not a possibility; we return to experience it all again.

The highest levels of consciousness belong to individuals who came to teach, such as Jesus/Yeshua Christ, Buddha, Paramahamsa Yogananda, Alara Kalama, and some species in the animal kingdom, which vibrate at the highest levels of consciousness.

When a child is born, their level of consciousness is in a high state. The child is happy and does not hold a grudge. The child reveals its innate intelligence, knowing that it can walk and talk. The child learns everything about the humans around it and begins to learn from them through its own innate intelligence. This reveals from the beginning that we are born intelligent. We are not given intelligence by man or books. The brain is a recording machine; intelligence is who we are.

When a baby attempts to stand and fails the first few times, I have never heard a baby say, "Oh, I give up, get me a pram, I can't be bothered to stand or walk." The message of "can" and "cannot" comes from the human storyteller. The infant's innate intelligence is often buried by the programmes of its parents or caregivers.

Animals' levels of consciousness are evident in those who kill to survive. When animals reach a level of 200 or more, they no longer kill, transitioning from meat-eaters to non-meat-eaters. Grazing animals calibrate/vibrate at higher levels than 85% of humans. This mirrors human levels of consciousness: killing, controlling, imprisoning, and abusing occur as part of the ego's survival in low levels of consciousness.

What we have learned about ourselves has been an indoctrination, primarily from various religions. For example, the Nag Hammadi Scriptures in Egypt were hidden from early Christians. It was believed that Amun Ra's quotes were written in the Bible; however, Amun Ra is not the creator of all. He is considered a god of evil and the one who ordered man to say "Amen." Nevertheless, it is the premise that all light shall reveal the truth, and the truth shall set you free. Human beings contain a piece of God within us; this is called Gnosticism, and physical matter is subject to decay and death. Humans are not the body-mind; this body is our vehicle.

The murder, rape, and pillage in Jabesh-Gilead are described in the King James Bible (31:17–18):

"Now therefore kill every male among the little ones, and kill every woman that hath known man by lying with him, but all the woman children that hath not known a man by lying with him, keep alive for yourselves."

If a man is caught raping a young girl, he must pay 50 pieces to her father and marry her (imagine a child having to marry her rapist), and he is not allowed to divorce her… and all is forgiven.

We have been told mostly how bad we are and how to become good, rather than how good we are and how our lived experiences and wrong beliefs shape us. We then develop an intention.

The Expectancy Theory, also known as the Expectancy Theory of Motivation, suggests that individuals choose a particular behaviour over others because they are motivated by the expected outcome of that behaviour. Essentially, the decision to engage in a certain behaviour is influenced by how desirable the outcome is perceived to be. Nevertheless, the theory emphasises the cognitive process through which individuals evaluate various motivational factors before making a final decision. It highlights that the outcome alone is not the only factor that determines behaviour (Victor Vroom, 1964).

The Mind

Homeostasis

A balance in all the body's systems is necessary for its correct function and existence. The whole body is a mind, and we inhabit it. It is our house, furnished with everything it needs to keep us happy and healthy. It loves us so much that it will adjust itself to always do the best it can for us, even when we do not treat it well, both inside and out.

Psychological Junk Food

We are told who we are, but we are not asked who we are. We determine our identity based on being programmed into a set of labels and stories. These labels and stories are our interpretations of our experiences and what we have absorbed—both negatively and positively—from those around us. The information we take in from the world around us is what we use to form a character, and we believe we are that character. But we are behind the character. Who is the thinker?

My studies in psychotherapy and my work as an Eye Movement Desensitization and Reprocessing (EMDR) therapist and psychotherapist have led me to a continuous study of human beings and how we are impacted by the constructs that have shaped—and continue to shape—us and our environment.

Some of the thoughts my clients share with me are horrific, derogatory, harsh, hateful, damning, greedy, jealous, and abusive. I recognise that we do not plan within ourselves to think these thoughts; rather, they arise in us because of the environment we grew up in. I often ask my clients: *Would you ever plan these thoughts?*

For example, would you say to yourself, *Tomorrow, I am going to think about myself in a horrific way,* or *I am going to plan to tell myself a horrible story to incite fear in myself until it creates such a fearful narrative that my body will respond with a sensation in my chest or stomach—an energy that has been labelled as the feeling of fear?*

At present, there are nearly eight billion people on the planet (or so I have been informed), each with their own story—unless they are babies or enlightened beings, which one might argue are the same, as a baby's programs are not yet fully formed.

Freud's Interpretation of the Structure in the Brain.

Freud postulated that an infant's foundational personality is set by the age of five to seven years, during which the child grasps how to survive in its environment. We are given an idea of who we are based on our experiences and what we are told about ourselves, but we are not asked.

Often, parents comment on their child's behaviour, saying: "I don't know where they got that behaviour from."

If the parent disapproves of the child's behaviour, they might attribute it to the other parent, saying, "He/she is just like their father" or "He/she is just like their mother," whether the behaviour is negative or positive.

The rest of a child's development appears to be shaped by their actions, reactions, and interpretations of who they believe they are or how they should act, based on the world around them.

The Chatter in Your Head

The question of who is responsible for the constant chatter in our minds can be answered by understanding that the brain appears to function as a recording machine. I specifically say *the brain in your head* because I believe the whole body is a brain.

Freud's theory of the **id, ego, and superego** illustrates this concept:

1. **The id** – The part of the personality driven by pleasure and the avoidance of pain.

2. **The ego** – The mediator between the id and the superego.

3. **The superego** – The moralistic part of the personality that enforces judgments of right and wrong.

Together, these three components form what we call egoistic thinking. This thinking is a phenomenon of constructed narratives—stories we have gathered from our environment. These influences include parents, caregivers, extended family members, teachers, and society. The brain functions like a recording device, replaying these stories repeatedly. These external influences shape our sense of self, even though they are not truly who we are.

The **egoic voice** is the one that believes it is always right, superior, and the centre of the universe. We give this voice our full attention, obeying its commands without realising that it is merely a recording of past experiences, societal messages, and beliefs about who we think we are.

But these are not *who you are*. The egoic voice is an idealised, made-up identity—a schizophrenic voice, endlessly repeating its story. And yet, you listen, as if it is telling you something new every time.

This repetitive narrative **activates energy in your body**, causing you to feel the same emotions over and over again. You become trapped in a cycle of repeated thoughts and feelings, reacting to this story as if it defines you. However, the story never actually speaks of *you*—it only speaks of your experiences, what others have said to you, and how your body-mind has reacted.

The Human-Doing

You have falsely believed that you are this *human-doing* because you have been programmed to work, comply, and please others. This is what previous generations have taught you because it is what they, too, learned and experienced in their lives.

Hence the saying: *Hurt people, hurt people.*

But still, *you have not met yourself.* You have been buried under all these stories. The real *you* existed before your mind was ever programmed.

I have not met a client who tells me who they truly are. Instead, they tell me about their stories—stories based on the teachings, beliefs, and experiences of others. They have built a character of themselves based on these external influences.

But the character is *not* who you are; it is who you *act as.*

We then repeat this cycle and pass it on to the next generation. We express and relive our experiences, suffering because we believe we *are* those experiences.

We develop an intimate relationship with our past experiences, recreating them in the present. This becomes our unfinished business—a repetition of childhood beliefs and experiences that we continue to carry into adulthood. Many people cling to the fantasy that *the world needs to change in order to make them feel better.*

But *we are not this.*

We pass on what we have learned, but is what we have learned **true**?

This cycle manifests physically, mentally, and emotionally. Many people develop narcissistic tendencies, blaming the world and believing the world owes them something. This mindset often plays out in relationships—someone says they love another, and in return, they expect love back. However, this expectation often stems from unresolved issues within themselves, placing the burden of their emotional healing onto another person.

John. N. Mitchell, quote;

"Our attitude towards life determines, life's attitude toward us".

Erich Fromm's professional journey spanned from the 1920s to the 1970s, during which he established himself as a sociologist and psychoanalyst. Fromm articulated that mental health equates to adjustment, suggesting that it is merely the state of not being more unwell than the average individual.

He proposed that this notion has been diminished to align with the prevailing societal level of discontent, leading individuals to avoid standing out from the general population. Furthermore, many contemporary definitions of mental health revolve around the absence of illness, where sickness is perceived as a failure to adjust or is characterised by specific symptoms such as alcoholism or insomnia. However, Fromm defined mental health not simply as the absence of illness but in a more affirmative context, emphasising wellness—a state that is often rare and overlooked.

In discussing mental health, Fromm asserted that a productive society would ultimately disintegrate if individuals were unaware of their mental illnesses. The challenge arises when individuals remain oblivious to their conditions, often deceiving themselves through various means of escape.

Fromm contended that a significant number of individuals deemed 'normal' may be more troubled than those labelled as neurotic, as the former are often unaware of their symptoms. Society tends to define normalcy based on shared experiences, leading to a situation where the norm itself becomes a form of sickness. This is exacerbated by a culture that provides numerous distractions and avenues for escape.

He observed that if individuals were left alone without the distractions that feed their egoic thoughts—such as radio, alcohol, cigarettes, or other diversions—they would likely experience numerous nervous breakdowns. He noted that the many escape routes available under the guise of fun, pleasure, food, and leisure often cause people to lose touch with their deeper humanity, resulting in a profound forgetfulness of their true selves.

Fromm argued that much of what individuals perceive about their well-being is a mere illusion, often influenced by the medications they take or by their attempts to escape reality through alcohol, drugs, entertainment, or obsessive behaviours. People frequently seek distractions outside themselves, making their claims about personal well-being unreliable.

A truly healthy individual, Fromm suggested, possesses clarity and awareness in their responses to the world, characterised by a lack of egocentrism. This person can realistically experience both the world and themselves as they truly are, responding authentically to their surroundings.

When asked whether American society is realistic, Fromm responded:

"I believe we are likely the most unrealistic societies that have ever existed."

He argued that we deceive ourselves regarding love, aspirations, and individuality, while in reality, we are constantly conforming. This phenomenon is evident in our reaction to the existential threat of global self-destruction.

Fromm's critique extends beyond America to encompass the entire world. He likened the situation to a scenario in which a bomb, capable of killing thousands, is carelessly handled: *"Everyone is aware of the threat to human life that we have normalised, and if that does not signify a lack of realism, I am uncertain what does."*

Fromm refers here to anyone involved in the creation of such bombs. What kind of person—man or woman—engages in such work in the first place, showing a blatant disregard for human life, no matter what justification we attempt to construct?

This lack of realism pertains not only to warfare but also to the production and consumption of goods. In our obsession with these processes, both production and consumption continue to escalate. Unbeknownst to us, we transform into mere objects, losing our individuality despite frequent discussions about it.

We follow leaders who fail to provide genuine guidance, believing we are acting on our own impulses, convictions, and opinions. In reality, we are manipulated by an entire industry driven by slogans, leaving us without any true purpose. As a result, we become alienated from our true selves.

The essence of our pursuit is not to stand out, yet we are paralysed by fear. We have deluded ourselves regarding the reality of our incessant discussions about our traditional heritage.

Fromm argued that a significant peril exists within the fields of psychology, psychoanalysis, and psychiatry, particularly concerning those who aim to assist individuals in conforming more effectively to societal expectations. This could lead psychology to become a mere facilitator of industrial systems, where individuals are conditioned to produce and consume en masse, often under the influence of centralised slogans.

Simultaneously, people remain oblivious to their dissatisfaction—a condition the French in the 18th century termed ennui, or boredom stemming from the meaninglessness of existence. The risk here is that individuals may develop psychological ailments, expressing their discontent and striving for a more meaningful life.

In response, many psychologists might argue that such dissatisfaction indicates neurosis, suggesting that individuals should be adjusted to accept a life devoid of meaning, without any form of rebellion or symptomatic expression.

Throughout history, numerous societies have exhibited signs of insanity, and we too may fall into this state unless a significant change occurs. There are two interpretations of sanity: one perspective views a society as sane if it conforms to its own norms, while it may simultaneously be deemed insane in a universal context regarding what is beneficial for humanity.

The great moral codes—whether derived from the Ten Commandments, the teachings of Jesus Christ, or the principles of Buddhism—represent standards of human sanity that pertain to the essence of human existence.

The principles that guide humanity are fundamentally rooted in the belief that loyalty to individuals and the values inherent in humanity surpass any allegiance to specific societies and their corresponding values.

Those who possess sound judgment and the bravery to voice their convictions align themselves with that segment of humanity—both in the present and historically—that is characterised by a remarkable trait: the ability to be a realist. This entails recognising the truth while simultaneously maintaining hope and not succumbing to despair.

"The fact that millions of people share the same vices does not make the vices a virtue, the fact that they share so many errors does not make the errors to be true, and the fact that millions of people share the same forms of mental pathology does not make these people sane."

Erich Fromm. (1955).

Fromm (1955) proposed that there are five fundamental human needs:

1. **Relatedness**
2. **Transcendence**
3. **Rootedness**
4. **Sense of identity**
5. **Frame of orientation**

Narcissism

Individuals who have not transcended (grown out of) primary narcissism frequently find themselves withdrawing from others and society. This behaviour stems from their failure to progress beyond an infantile stage, leading them to perceive the world subjectively, primarily in terms of fulfilling their own needs.

From this perspective, the people surrounding them are regarded merely as objects whose purpose is to provide nourishment, comfort, and care, rather than as distinct individuals. Consequently, they lack an objective view of others. However, if an infant is nurtured in a supportive environment, they can move beyond primary narcissism, recognising others as meaningful individuals. This development fosters the capacity to love and acknowledge that the needs of others hold equal significance to their own.

As noted by Fromm (1955) and Freud (1944), *"Narcissism is the essence of all severe psychic pathology."* The narcissist exists within a reality shaped solely by their own thoughts, emotions, and desires, failing to engage with the external world in an objective manner.

Those who have not overcome their fixation on their mother often develop a sense of helplessness or a victim mentality. This neurotic state is driven by a subconscious fantasy: *if I am the helpless child, then my mother will come to take care of me.*

However, as adults, they may submit to a group that appears to offer them comfort but instead exploits them to advance its own agenda, fostering a mob mentality. This can lead to an excessive attachment to a sense of national identity rather than recognising oneself as a child of a greater creator, as all humans are. Their perception of those they deem as 'alien' or a 'threat' becomes distorted due to societal divisions created by labels and traditions.

Relatedness

Relatedness provides insight into individuals considered to be insane, as such people have not succeeded in establishing a cohesive relationship with themselves, thereby remaining trapped within their own psyche. A genuine connection is formed when an individual engages meaningfully with others.

Many people find themselves in **symbiotic relationships**, which are often characterised by a dynamic between a submissive individual and a sadistic partner. These individuals depend on each other to attain a sense of wholeness, yet they remain ensnared in their own limitations, failing to evolve into healthy individuals.

This type of unhealthy relationship acts as a coping mechanism to evade the challenges associated with freedom. The essence of a symbiotic relationship is rooted in one person's self-worth being contingent upon the other. In contrast, authentic love within a relationship is defined by both individuals maintaining their integrity and individuality.

Loving oneself and others entails recognising and accepting separateness, enabling each person to remain true to their identity without the need to change themselves to meet the expectations of the other.

Thus, the ultimate choice for humankind, as we are driven to transcend ourselves, is to create or destroy, to love or to hate.

Rootedness

Every adult requires help, warmth, and protection, much like a child. However, an adult's sense of rootedness is more connected to the external world rather than solely to a mother or caregiver.

The similarity lies in the way adults feel grounded within society, often through affiliations such as religion or tribal identity. This sense of belonging can lead to the formation of homogeneous groups, where those who do not share the same qualities or beliefs are perceived as alien or even as threats.

However, in seeking a sense of identity, an individual may find comfort and stability in rootedness but also feel trapped by it— unable to step out of their comfort zone, or what has long ceased to be comfortable. This incestuous fixation on a homogeneous group distorts one's relationship with the self, the group, and outsiders. When an individual has not yet fully developed into a complete human being, they remain bound in a psychological prison, crippled by their own need for security, which can lead to mental instability.

Those who become psychologically unwell are often disconnected from nature and instead construct their identity through imagination and reasoning—defining themselves by labels such as *"I am this"* or *"I am that."* This phenomenon is even more pronounced in modern society, where the need for a strong identity has become a driving force, shaping false beliefs about the self. Many individuals seek validation through status, fame, gender identity, or ideological affiliation, rather than embracing a more organic sense of being.

A person begins to approach reality only when they look at the world as it truly is and gradually strip away illusions and trivialities. The more an individual explores a frame of orientation—which can include spirituality—the closer they come to understanding reality. However, this exploration can also be deceptive if it merely satisfies the individual's need for meaning rather than offering genuine insight.

Fromm described this as mankind's tendency to understand the world through thought rather than intelligence. Thought is often used as a tool to manipulate reality, whereas intelligence, which arises from the *human* aspect of our nature, allows for deeper comprehension. These two forces—reason (rooted in our animal instincts) and intelligence (rooted in our human nature)—are often in conflict.

The Need for a Frame of Orientation

The need for a frame of orientation exists on two levels.

1. **Fundamental Need:** Every person requires some form of orientation, regardless of whether it is true or false. Without

a subjectively satisfying framework, an individual cannot maintain a stable existence.

2. **Engagement with Reality:** The second level involves the necessity to engage with reality through reason, allowing for an objective understanding of the world.

However, the need to establish a frame of orientation is often more urgent than the drive to cultivate reason, as it directly impacts an individual's sense of happiness and tranquility rather than their mental stability. This is particularly evident in the role of rationalisation.

Many individuals who are perceived as intelligent may still become trapped in harmful environments or organisations due to their overwhelming need for a structured worldview. This need often outweighs their ability to think critically. As a result, even highly educated people may endorse flawed ideas or engage in detrimental behaviours, simply because their sense of belonging and purpose depends on it.

"Mental health is achieved if man develops into full maturity according to the characteristics and the laws of human nature. Mental illness consists in a failure of such development. From this premise, the criterion of mental health is not one of individual adjustment to a given social order, but a universal one, valid for all men, of giving a satisfactory answer to the problem of human existence." — Erich Fromm (1955).

The Power of Belief: Dr Bruce Lipton's Perspective

Dr Bruce Lipton explores the connection between conscious thought and the biochemical composition of our blood. He explains that negative thoughts can trigger the release of harmful substances into the bloodstream, adversely affecting physical well-being. Conversely, positive thoughts stimulate the secretion of beneficial biochemicals, promoting cellular vitality and overall health. This dynamic plays a significant role in shaping genetic expression.

This concept has long been recognised in medicine as the placebo effect—the phenomenon in which a person's expectation of a positive outcome influences their actual experience.

For example, Lipton describes a case where a physician prescribes a *new purple pill* to a patient suffering from an ailment. The patient, believing in the pill's effectiveness, begins to recover— only to later discover that the pill was nothing more than a sugar tablet. The key factor in their recovery was not the pill itself but the patient's belief in its power.

This response is rooted in societal conditioning, which teaches individuals from a young age to place trust in medical professionals and external solutions rather than in their own capacity for healing.

Ultimately, belief is a powerful force. A positive belief system fosters beneficial biochemical responses, leading to biological transformation. Conversely, negative beliefs can generate stress and emotional distress, directly influencing our mood and well-being.

In conclusion, our perceptions—shaped by belief—can either heal us or harm us. The mind's influence over the body is profound, demonstrating that mental health is not just a matter of external circumstances but also of internal conviction.

The Creation of a Human-Doing (The Slave).

Nursery - Separation anxiety.

When nursing your baby, you might be advised to let them cry for extended periods before responding. This approach is intended to train the child, but it often does more harm than good, particularly for the baby. Instead of fostering independence, it teaches the child that their parent or caregiver is unavailable to meet their needs, which can lead to separation anxiety.

A child's cries are not a sign of being spoiled or manipulative; rather, they are a natural expression of their need for connection, safety, and love—essential elements for healthy development. Just as adults instinctively recognise their hunger, babies have an innate understanding of their emotional needs that only their caregivers can truly address.

The baby and the parent share a bonding experience, which is expressed through non-verbal communication, known as intersubjectivity and musicality.

The Importance of Touch in Early Development

For a baby, touch is a fundamental form of communication. Skin-to-skin contact is essential not only for regulating body temperature but also for normal physiological and emotional development. When a baby lacks sufficient physical contact with a parent or caregiver, they may become angry, anxious, or frustrated.

Babies who are deprived of touch fail to thrive, and in severe cases, may stop growing altogether. A lack of physical contact can also impact the myelination of a baby's nerves, affecting brain development. Throughout life, touch remains an important part of human communication, helping us connect, feel safe, and relieve stress.

In many cases, when infants cry or show discomfort, parents or caregivers instinctively put something in the infant's mouth or hand to distract them. However, this often reflects the caregiver's own preoccupation with personal addictions—whether to devices, substances, or other compulsive behaviours—resulting in the infant's needs being neglected. In this way, children learn that these addictions take precedence over their well-being.

What we do to ourselves, we do to those around us. This becomes apparent when a frustrated parent tells a child, *"You're getting on my nerves,"* when in reality, it is their own mental overload that is overwhelming them, leaving little room for the child's needs.

Who Are the Savages?

Dr Gabor Maté experienced trauma and separation anxiety as a child when he was taken from his parents to save his life from Adolf Hitler's reign of ethnic cleansing.

Maté raises critical questions about the nature of wealth accumulation, suggesting that it often stems from selfishness—an attitude instilled by society. He challenges whether this behaviour is truly inherent to human nature and explores the developmental needs of children.

Maté argues that a child's well-being is significantly influenced by whether their emotional needs are met. He observes that in many cultures, parents maintain close physical contact with their infants, while in Western societies, children are often separated from their parents—placed in prams, sent to childcare, or left to cry without comfort, sometimes on the advice of midwives or nursery staff.

This approach contrasts sharply with the nurturing practices of other cultures, where children are comforted in times of distress.

The Impact of a Fast-Paced Society on Parenting

In today's fast-paced, consumer-driven world, time is a scarce resource. Many parents, bound by demanding schedules, prioritise their own needs over those of their children. In contrast, traditional indigenous communities in Africa and the Americas have historically kept their infants close at all times, guided by natural parenting instincts.

Babies cry because it is their only way of communicating stress. When an infant cry for their parent, it is not an act of *tyranny*—it is an expression of a fundamental need for emotional and physical connection.

The Ferber method (Ferberisation), introduced by Richard Ferber in 2006, is one of many techniques that promote sleep training through controlled crying. While widely accepted in Western parenting, such methods often overlook the essential developmental requirements of a child.

Western societies frequently encourage parents to let their babies cry without comfort. However, in many cultures, children are instinctively soothed when they cry. Scientific research shows that leaving a child to cry alone elevates cortisol levels, inducing stress—just as it would for any individual left in distress without support.

The Consequences of Emotional Deprivation

Harry Harlow's disturbing 1960 experiment on infant monkeys demonstrated that, when given a choice between a wire mother providing food and a soft, comforting mother figure, the monkeys overwhelmingly preferred the nurturing presence, even at the expense of food.

Similar findings have been observed in feral children—those who have grown up with extreme neglect. Their psychological and emotional development is significantly impaired due to the lack of human connection during their early years.

Despite such evidence, medical models have historically advocated methods like Ferberisation, encouraging parents to let infants cry rather than responding to their needs.

Stress and Intergenerational Trauma

Maté explains how stress is transmitted from one generation to the next. A child cannot self-regulate; they mirror their parent's emotional state. If a parent is stressed, the child absorbs this stress, leading to difficulties in emotional regulation. This cycle continues when the child grows up and becomes a parent themselves.

Maté critiques the Western tendency to dissociate the mind from the body, a division that increases susceptibility to illness. Stress has profound physiological effects, particularly on the lungs, contributing to conditions such as asthma.

The disconnection from parents and family during childhood is deeply damaging to human well-being. This concept has been recognised for centuries and is reflected in the interconnectedness observed in nature and Buddhist philosophy.

Maté also challenges the medical approach of treating conditions like asthma and inflammation with steroids, which are synthetic versions of **cortisol**, the body's stress hormone. He argues that stress is embedded in our lives from birth—through family separation, over-medication, and increasing dependence on technology.

The Role of Technology and Consumerism

Excessive mobile phone use and other digital distractions often lead to the neglect of children's emotional needs. As a result, consumerism takes precedence over human relationships.

As society becomes more reliant on technology, genuine human connection is diminishing. This growing disconnection exacerbates stress, further perpetuating cycles of neglect and emotional deprivation.

In prioritising wealth, convenience, and external validation over meaningful relationships, we risk losing what is most essential: the deep, instinctive bonds that form the foundation of healthy emotional and psychological development.

Consequently, this environment of stress can result in withdrawal behaviours in both adults and children, as they seek to shield themselves from feelings of abandonment. Such dynamics elevate cortisol levels, which can trigger autoimmune diseases and mental health issues.

The First Prison.

The Prison that induces stress, anxiety, and, above all, separation anxiety from a very early age is the mandatory institution you are compelled to attend. Your separation anxiety is disregarded and normalised by a society conditioned to prioritise productivity over emotional well-being.

You are not free to leave at will, you must consume the provided food, and you are constantly reminded that you are not good enough (if you haven't already received that message at home). You may have been instructed to improve and told that you lack confidence, effort, or diligence.

It is absurd to expect you to acquire these qualities as if they were commodities readily available for purchase. You are doing your best with the experiences, emotions, and psychological challenges you are facing.

You are required to wear the designated uniform, but what will you truly learn?

You will learn to conform to the invisible regulations of society, such as *should*, *must*, and *have to*. We are left with an undercurrent of fear. These rules will shape your entire life, conditioning you to conform to the prevailing culture. You will become a mere executor of tasks, without being taught anything about your true essence as a human being.

What is this confining institution called? It is known as school or nursery.

You have done nothing wrong, yet you will be forcibly separated from your family—by your own family—as they adhere to the unspoken rules of society.

You will have to navigate the unresolved issues of all the adults in the nursery or school. Teachers, acting as prison guards, will enforce these rules, whether they are healthy or unhealthy. If you do not comply, you will be punished.

Teachers are often influenced by their own unconscious programming from childhood, shaped by the negative behaviours they absorbed from their early life experiences at home and in school.

This is what we call learning to socialise.

We exist in a constant state of survival, learning how to appease those who came before us—whether they are adults or children whom we perceive as threatening or formidable.

The Second Prison

Individuals who find themselves incarcerated are essentially expressing the culmination of their upbringing, the beliefs instilled in them, and their perception of self—just like all of us.

This expression manifests through emotions such as anger, pain, abuse, rage, guilt, and cruelty, among others.

However, this prison is not confined within the physical walls of a jail cell; rather, it resides within the repetitive narrative of our own egotistical minds. It is akin to living in a perpetual loop, reliving the same experiences over and over—much like the film *Groundhog Day*.

Even when we believe we have undergone a transformation, such as transitioning from poverty to wealth, our past experiences can still dictate our actions as we strive to prove our worthiness. If you still harbour feelings of inadequacy and possess an insatiable drive for more, you may recognise this pattern within yourself.

This phenomenon is often observed in individuals who excel in their professional lives but struggle to form meaningful relationships, finding it challenging to connect with others.

Those trapped in this cycle frequently attempt to fill the void through excessive spending and self-gratification.

"You should not feel bad for the guilt that others project onto you,

You should feel grateful for recognising that it is their projection"

Isabell Thomas (2024).

Child and Animal Experiments

Attachment theory.

In the 1950s and 1960s, psychological research was dominated by psychoanalysts and behaviourists. John B. Watson was considered a pioneering psychologist. After graduating in 1908, Watson began teaching psychology and observing human behaviours. His work fell under the realm of natural science, which deals with the physical world.

However, the experiments that Watson carried out demonstrated that, in this instance—and many others—natural science does not adequately address human beings. His doctrine was aimed at prediction and control (Watson, 1913).

Many behavioural experiments were conducted with some form of cruelty, either towards animals or humans. For example, Harry

Harlow (1965) used monkeys to explore whether infants loved their parents or were only interested in their mothers for food.

Harlow conducted an experiment on infant monkeys by removing them from their mothers at birth. The monkeys were isolated in cages for varying durations—some for three months, others for six months, and some for up to a year. This experiment had a detrimental and devastating impact on the infant monkeys, particularly those kept in isolation for the longest periods.

When these monkeys were later introduced to others, those who had been isolated the longest would hold themselves and rock back and forth. They were often so distressed that they would mutilate themselves. They also became aggressive towards each other. When these monkeys later became parents, they displayed severe deficits in caregiving, attacking and even killing their own offspring (Blum, 2011).

A similarly unethical experiment was carried out on an eight-month-old infant known as "Little Albert"—though this was not the child's real name. Watson and his graduate assistant, Rosalie Rayner (1920), conducted an experiment based on classical conditioning on a little boy named Douglas Merritte.

Douglas was placed in close proximity to various objects, including a monkey, a dog, a rabbit, and a white rat. At first, he explored the objects and appeared to enjoy interacting with the white rat. However, the experiment began when Watson introduced a distressing stimulus. Every time Douglas touched the white rat, he was subjected to a loud bang—a hammer striking a metal bar.

This process was repeated until Douglas became visibly distressed. As a result, he not only developed a conditioned fear of furry animals but also began to fear fur itself, as seen when he reacted negatively to Watson wearing a Santa Claus mask.

Watson wanted to determine whether this conditioned fear would persist over time, so he instructed that Douglas be brought back a month later to repeat the experiment. The results confirmed that Douglas retained the fear Watson had instilled in him.

Furthermore, the name change to "Little Albert" may have been an attempt to conceal Douglas Merritte's true identity. While he was initially presented as a healthy child, records indicate that he suffered from hydrocephalus, a medical condition that ultimately led to his death at the age of six.

Bowlby's Attachment Theory

John Bowlby's (1988) work as a child psychiatrist was heavily influenced by ethological theory, particularly Lorenz's (1970) study on imprinting. Lorenz demonstrated that attachment is an innate behaviour in young ducklings and serves a survival purpose.

Bowlby proposed that both infants and mothers have evolved a biological need to stay in contact with each other. He argued that infants who remained close to their mothers had a higher chance of survival and reproduction.

In line with his evolutionary theory of attachment, Bowlby believed that attachment behaviours, such as seeking proximity, are instinctive and are triggered by any circumstances that threaten closeness—such as separation, insecurity, or fear. He also suggested that the fear of strangers is an important survival mechanism inherent in humans from birth.

Bowlby argued that children are biologically predisposed to form attachments, as this is crucial for their survival. He introduced the concept of primary attachment, or monotropy, which refers to the unique and qualitatively different bond that a child forms with one primary caregiver.

According to Bowlby, there is a critical period—around 2.5 years—for attachment development. If an attachment does not form during this period, it may never occur. However, he later proposed a sensitive period of up to five years, during which attachment can still develop, though with greater difficulty.

Bowlby's maternal deprivation hypothesis suggests that consistent disruption of the attachment between an infant and their primary caregiver can lead to long-term cognitive, social, and emotional difficulties.

Additionally, Bowlby introduced the concept of an internal working model—a cognitive framework that consists of mental representations for understanding the world, oneself, and others. This model, shaped by the child's relationship with their primary caregiver, serves as a prototype for future social relationships. It enables individuals to predict, control, and navigate their interactions with others.

These attachment behaviours are akin to fixed action patterns and influence an infant's interactions with others. The infant exhibits innate 'social releaser' behaviours, such as crying and smiling, to elicit caregiving from adults. The key factor in attachment is not food but rather care and responsiveness.

Additional attachments may form in a hierarchical manner. An infant may have a primary monotropy attachment to the mother, followed by attachments to the father, siblings, grandparents, and so on. Bowlby posits that this initial attachment is fundamentally distinct from extended ones, such as those formed with society, emphasising the unique nature of the relationship with the mother.

Bowlby also highlighted the critical period for attachment formation, suggesting that maternal care delayed beyond certain timeframes could have long-lasting effects on the child. Maternal deprivation, as described by Bowlby, encompasses separation, loss, or failure to establish an attachment with the mother.

The concept of monotropy, as proposed by Bowlby, underscores the importance of a strong bond with a single attachment figure, warning of potential negative outcomes if this bond is disrupted. Bowlby's maternal deprivation hypothesis stemmed from his theory of monotropy. He believed that the relationship between an infant and mother in the first five years of life played a crucial role in socialisation.

According to Bowlby, if separation from the primary caregiver occurs during the critical period (birth to five years old) without adequate emotional care, the child may face significant challenges.

Bowlby initially believed that the consequences of deprivation were irreversible and would have long-term effects on a child's intellectual, social, and emotional development. These effects included delinquency, reduced intelligence, increased aggression, depression, and affectionless psychopathy.

Bowlby argued that the absence of emotional care could result in affectionless psychopathy, which is characterised by a lack of concern for others, a lack of guilt, and an inability to form meaningful relationships.

Individuals with affectionless psychopathy often act impulsively without considering the consequences of their actions, such as showing no remorse for antisocial behaviour. Bowlby concluded that maternal deprivation during a child's early life caused permanent emotional harm.

Isabell Thomas

Social Programming
from Entertainment.

It is apparent in society and through my work that media programming plays a significant role in shaping beliefs about the world and ourselves. It is also clear to me that the world is made up of stories that we have the choice to believe once we become aware of them. However, some stories have become deeply ingrained in our lives, leading to their normalisation in society—essentially, believing in made-up narratives.

Shakespeare famously wrote:

"All the world's a stage, and all the men and women merely players."

This reflects how mental illness is often normalised as typical behaviour. For example, I remember watching Disney films as a child, and I loved them. They felt comforting, evoked a sense of well-being, and gave me a feel-good factor. However, over time, I began to see them differently—like a version of *Hansel and Gretel*.

They seemed to be telling another story beneath the surface. As many children do, I asked, "Is this real?" The answer was, *"No, darling, it's made up."* I asked the same question when something on TV scared me and received the same response. While I understood it was a fictional story, I also realised it was one that we, as a society, choose to believe.

42

This is why I compare it to *Hansel and Gretel*—like the fairy tale, these films lure us into something that appears sweet, innocent, and inviting, but beneath the surface, it can be something quite different.

In therapy, this is known as 'unfinished business'—an unresolved issue from childhood that continues to play out in one's life. Take, for example, *Beauty and the Beast*. The story follows the turmoil of a man capturing a young woman because he desires her, with his fellow males agreeing—depicted through the singing and dancing in the film.

We see narcissism in both Gaston and, initially, the Beast. Belle's father is then captured by the Beast, who trades him for Belle. Over time, Belle begins to develop feelings for the Beast (Stockholm Syndrome), and eventually, the spell is broken, transforming the Beast into a prince (a 'good person'), leading to the classic happily-ever-after.

Stories like this play out in adulthood because they have influenced our minds. How many children and adults dream of being a princess and say, *"I want the fairy tale"*? This concept is reflected in the traditional wedding dress, or in phrases such as, *"I will treat you like a princess"* or *"I should be treated like a princess."* This has led to what is sometimes called 'princess syndrome' in both men and women.

Men are often depicted as the 'beast,' reinforcing the idea that staying in an abusive relationship will eventually lead to change—that, like in the film, the person will magically transform.

Certain men, women, and teenagers have become the subjects of sexual objectification, often driven by an ego-| admiration for their own sexualisation. They may feel compelled to engage in sexual activities in particular ways to satisfy male or female partners.

Conversely, some men may believe they are entitled to act in certain ways, viewing such behaviour as acceptable even when it causes harm and trauma to their partners. This lack of awareness stems from societal norms that have normalised these behaviours in both males and females.

In the film *Maurice*, the character is portrayed as insane and powerless due to his age and inability to protect his daughter. This leads him to accept his troubling fate, reinforcing the idea that he is no longer needed in society—a concept often referred to as a 'mid-life crisis'. But could this be the result of early psychological programming?

This narrative also reflects broader societal issues regarding the exploitation of children. Additionally, men who experience abuse may remain silent, constrained by societal expectations of masculinity that obscure the impact of their childhood experiences—including the influence of a harmful maternal figure.

Seeking Help, Outside of the Mainstream.

The human brain is an extraordinary organ. From the onset of our existence, it operates at specific frequencies of brain waves that facilitate our growth and development. For instance, during the first year of life, an infant's brain predominantly exhibits Delta waves, characterised by a low frequency ranging from 0.1 to 3.5 Hz. Delta waves are associated with the sleep state, a period when we detach from the external physical world and are instead drawn inward by the compelling sensation of sleep.

This state also represents the domain of our unconscious mind, which retains essential aspects of what we have learned and experienced from our surroundings.

The subsequent brainwave frequency is Theta, which ranges from 4 to 8 Hz. This frequency is believed to be present in children up to the age of 13 while they are awake. Theta is often regarded as a reflection of our limbic system, as the activity within this frequency is where information from our surroundings is processed and stored.

It encompasses our experiences, memories, emotions, feelings, and actions. This frequency is particularly evident when a child is daydreaming and is integral to our intuition, creativity, and imagination. This state is crucial for our understanding of the environment and represents the sleep or unconscious state that we frequently experience, regardless of whether we are children or adults.

Growing up in an environment that is out of balance can heavily impact development. For a child who experiences a mixture of trauma, unhealthy dynamics, and some positive moments, these experiences can continue to play out in adulthood due to the influence of the Theta frequency.

For example, if a child or adult is reminded of past trauma through a trigger in the present moment, their reaction may stem from the unconscious mind operating in Theta frequency. This is often referred to as survival mode, where the person avoids situations to escape discomfort they have previously experienced. Avoidant behaviour can be a defence mechanism, and if a person is in a state of distress or dis-ease, their reactions may appear erratic or unusual.

We often follow, trust, and even worship those who vibrate at lower levels of consciousness. Because our consciousness is inherently aware of truth and lies, we respond physically and mentally. As a result, when we remain at these low levels, we experience mental and physical illness, unhappiness, and discomfort—essentially, a state akin to *Hell* on this level of consciousness.

The Alpha frequency, ranging between 8 to 12 Hz, represents a state in which we feel more present, with a sense of clarity and inner peace. In this state, tasks can be completed more effectively and efficiently, with ease. Within the Alpha frequency, we perceive the world around us more truthfully and experience a deeper sense of well-being.

It is understandable why ancient civilisations placed great importance on vibration as both a creative and destructive force, as well as a tool for healing—capable of eradicating diseased cells. Everything in the universe is a vibration, including our words. Positive words carry a vibration, just as negative words towards ourselves and others do, each possessing its own Hz frequency.

The first known use of music as a healing force comes from the Australian Aborigines—or should they be referred to as the *Origins?*—who have used the didgeridoo as a healing tool for more than 40,000 years. Similarly, Yogic and Chinese traditions incorporate certain spoken sounds, known as *bija*, into chants, mantras, and meditations targeting different parts of the body.

Chanting is particularly powerful in healing. It is believed to create an opiate-like effect in the body, which can help overcome both mental and physical pain and injury.

The Greeks also recognised music as a tool for healing. Pythagoras, often credited as a mathematician, was also known as the *Father of Music*. He discovered the mathematical beauty of harmonic intervals, linking specific sounds to a pure and comprehensible sensation that, in his words, could create *"soul adjustments"*.

Pythagoras used harmonies to induce sleep when needed and to energise his disciples through different musical arrangements, which were considered divine.

Moving forward to more recent history, in 1896, American doctors first identified a connection between sound and healing, noting that music could improve blood flow and enhance cognitive processes (Zeng, F.-G., Tang, Q., Dimitrijevic, A., Starr, A., Larky, J., & Blevins, N.H, 2011). Music therapy was also widely used in the 1940s to rehabilitate soldiers returning from World War II.

This paved the way for the development of sound wave therapy in the 1950s by pioneering British osteopath Sir Peter Guy Manners. He created the first machine designed to produce sound vibrations for healing. Placed directly over the affected body part and set to the frequency of healthy cells in that region, the device was believed to restore cells to their natural, healthy state. By the 1990s, Manners had developed the first computerised system capable of treating a range of conditions.

Following this, Dr Alfred Tomatis and Dr Guy Berard introduced auditory integration therapy, designed to improve conditions such as anxiety and learning disabilities.

More recently, scientific studies have begun investigating how sound can facilitate healing. Most research focuses on the release of *feel-good* chemicals in the brain's reward centres when listening to music or specific sounds. Although this field of study is still in its infancy, anecdotally, many people can confirm the profound effects of sound therapy.

The use of sound to treat ailments is both ancient and contemporary. While we are only beginning to understand the mechanisms behind these changes, our ancestors were already aware of the outcomes. They may not have been able to explain *how* sound worked, but they certainly knew *that* it worked.

Dr Lee Bartel discovered that insects tend to vibrate in harmony with the environment they are in. You may have heard of how a piano note can resonate with another piano in the same surroundings. Similarly, when entering a room, you can often sense its vibration—whether positive or negative. This is commonly expressed in phrases such as *"you could cut the tension with a knife."* Growing up in a negative vibrational environment may be experienced as a constant underlying sense of unease or nervous anticipation.

Dr Bartel suggests that music medicine operates at a low vibration of 7 Hz, which can positively impact cellular healing within the body.

He explains that when we hear a single click, the sound travels through the spine, affecting the cells via electrical signals that pass through the auditory nerves to the brain. The molecular compressions of sound, processed through the ear's hair cells in the cochlea, send vibrations via the auditory nerve to the brain. Alternatively, vibrations can also be detected through the skin, where mechanoreceptors translate them through the spinal cord to the brain, depending on the Hz frequency.

The relationship between beats per second and brain waves can be broken down as follows:

- **Delta:** 1 to 4 cycles per second (Hz)
- **Theta:** 4 to 8 cycles per second (Hz)
- **Alpha:** 8 to 12 cycles per second (Hz)
- **Beta:** 12 to 30 cycles per second (Hz)
- **Gamma:** 30 to 100 cycles per second (Hz)

When exposed to a consistent vibration, neurons synchronise their activity. This follows the principle that *"neurons that fire together wire together"*, impacting mood, motor function, pain perception, memory, and the limbic system.

Dr Bartel believes that the optimal healing vibration is 40 Hz. His research involved treating 18 patients with Alzheimer's disease using a 40 Hz vibration. The patients sat in a specialised chair equipped with speakers that transmitted the vibrations not only through sound but also through the air, allowing them to experience the frequency physically.

The patients used the chair for 30 minutes, two to three times per week. After just three weeks, improvements in memory were observed, with continued progress week after week. By the 12-week mark, patients showed significant memory recovery.

For those who wished to continue using vibration therapy beyond the initial 12-week period, the **Vibroacoustic Therapy System Plus VTS-2000** was made available. This technology may help slow the progression of Alzheimer's disease.

The Sun

Dr Jack Kruse, a neurosurgeon, made an intriguing discovery in 2017 regarding blue light toxins and their impact on weight gain. He found that exposure to light can trigger the production of certain chemicals in our bodies that were not present before. Additionally, Dr Kruse pointed out that many aspects of medicine are fundamentally misunderstood. He noted that the frequency of 7.8 Hz aligns with human brainwave activity.

The Earth's natural frequency, known as the Schumann Resonance, has drawn significant interest from scientists and researchers due to its potential health benefits. Energy enters through our eyes and is directed to the pineal gland, and it is essential to balance blue and red light to activate the pituitary gland. This insight led Dr Kruse to stop performing surgeries at 7 AM.

He believes that the answers to many health issues are right in front of us, but they can be obscured if dopamine levels are low. He explains that energy and mass are essentially the same, differing only by their environments. The public acts like a black box radiator, allowing light to enter and reflect back.

Moreover, all aromatic amino acids absorb ultraviolet light, and our eyes contain 23 different amino acids. The benzene ring functions as a photon trap, capturing UV light frequencies, which play a crucial role in biological processes. In 2014, Dr Kruse collaborated with Giuliano Preparata and others, discovering that 13% of the exclusion zone in water is completely coherent, equating to about 1 million free electrons. These delocalised electrons drive various biochemical functions, with around 100,000 processes occurring every second in a single cell.

The control of enzymatic activity is governed by molecular resonance phenomena, shedding light on the intricate workings of biochemistry.

Light is an electromagnetic wave that transforms into an electromechanical wave, known as sound, when it interacts with water. Water acts as a magnetic dipole, with hydrogen and oxygen carrying positive and negative charges, which is why it is associated with magnetism. This magnetism influences sound. When light penetrates water, it gets absorbed, altering the hydrogen bonding networks and potentially changing the water's density on a quantum level.

Mitochondria produce the cytosolic water that envelops various components within the cytosol, including the nucleus and mitochondria themselves. This connection arises from the interaction of sunlight with the Earth's ionosphere, often referred to as the Earth's heartbeat. This phenomenon creates an electrical tension between solar plasma and the atmosphere, generating a frequency of 7.83 Hz.

Dr Kruse discovered that the alpha wave in the human brain also resonates at 7.83 Hz, indicating that the solar system tunes us into these frequencies as they reach Earth, promoting the generation of alpha waves.

However, our current environment limits the number of alpha waves we experience. Non-native electromagnetic fields (EMF) can dehydrate our cells by reducing the redox potential in our mitochondria, meaning we produce less water from our mitochondria, leading to dehydration. This can be compared to cooking meat in a microwave, where the rapid rotation and vibration of water molecules dehydrate the meat, resulting in a tough texture. Similarly, our brains are affected by the toxic lifestyles we lead.

This process revolves around the eyes, with the suprachiasmatic nucleus (SCN) being the main focus, while in medicine, the spotlight is on the retina. This is why both young and elderly individuals visit the ophthalmologist for cataract surgery. After the surgery, they receive an implantable lens that blocks 100% of UV-A, UV-B, and UV-C rays, and currently, it also blocks 50% of blue light. Infrared light is balanced out by blue light, especially when the sun rises.

There are three types of solar radiation: UV-A, UV-B, and UV-C. However, they are not a threat since the ozone layer absorbs them, preventing harm to our eyes or vision. However, sources such as welding machines, tanning beds, and various lasers can produce harmful radiation.

What is crucial for our eyes is that blue light bends the most, which is significant because when it enters the eyes, it focuses in front of the retina. This can lead to vision issues as the eyeball elongates, resulting in myopia. Myopia can progress to retinal detachments and acute macular degeneration. Our eyes are not very effective at blocking blue light, so almost all visible blue light passes through the cornea and lens. This light is then processed by cells that convert it into images for the brain.

Continuous exposure to blue light can contribute to cataracts, eye cancer, and growths on the clear covering of the eye. A study from the National Eye Institute shows that children are at a higher risk than adults because they absorb more blue light from screens. By 2040, it is predicted that 288 million people will experience eye degeneration. Currently, around 1.5 million people in the UK are dealing with macular disease, affecting individuals of all ages.

Between 2003 and 2009, researchers discovered a new opsin in the eye called melanopsin, which works with retinal ganglion cells. This hormone plays a key role in the central retinal pathways, particularly at night, as it connects to melatonin production. The fovea, where most of the visual light spectrum is focused at the back of the eye, is often overlooked by many optometrists.

However, Japanese optometrists pay close attention to it because it relates to sharp vision. They understand that the central retinal pathways activate everything downstream, including the pituitary gland and various functions in the brain.

Professor Dr Fritz Hollwich, an ophthalmologist from Germany, made an interesting observation in 1909. He found that after removing cataracts without replacing the lens, patients could see UV light.

Additionally, back in 1891, neurosurgeon Santiago Ramón y Cajal documented energetic pathways that significantly impacted growth and metabolism through the eye. He noted that patients experienced better sleep, weight loss, and overall improved well-being after cataract surgery. Hollwich also experimented with animals and discovered that some changed colour, along with the presence of new metabolites in their urine post-surgery.

Kruse proposed the idea that light can actually form new chemicals in our bodies, linking back to Einstein's equation, $E=mc^2$. He suggests that light might transform into substances like melanosomes and melanin. This raises an important question: is it really just diet and exercise that keep us healthy?

Dr John Nash Ott found that light has the power to aid tissue regeneration. He observed that when plants were exposed to different types of light, their chloroplasts spun five times faster. Curious about this, he tested it on animals and discovered that the retinal pigment epithelium in the eye contains melanin granules that absorb UV light.

This absorption creates a direct current due to rapid movement, which helps regenerate the tissue nucleus when there is a strong electric current. However, excessive blue light can counteract vitamin A and DHA because it promotes the overproduction of vitamin A. Every opsin in our body is linked to retinol, and a lack of vitamin A is associated with obesity, diabetes, and mitochondrial issues. Kruse suggests that excess blue light contributes to weight gain.

Additionally, when light energy decreases, the pituitary gland enlarges, which can lead to weight gain as people tend to eat more. However, Kruse argues the opposite. When something is injured, it typically swells, suggesting that anything losing energy in the universe tends to expand. Hollwich pointed out that when light slows down, it transforms into hormones, which can alter nuclear DNA.

We produce melatonin in our eyes during the morning, and the hormone associated with darkness is also generated in the eyes. It is crucial to remember that our skin can also sense light and darkness, affecting hormone levels in our blood. In the morning, a mix of UVA and infrared A light is essential, and we should aim for more sunlight exposure during that time. Balancing blue and red light is important for hormone production.

Man-made UV light is harmful and disrupts how mitochondria process electrons from food. Kruse's insight is that "the laws of nature aren't influenced by human beliefs or experiments." We need more sunlight or heat, such as from a sauna, since infrared light is beneficial.

The Body

Why are we normalising cruelty?

I am of the belief that the entirety of the human body functions as a brain, communicating through intersubjectivity and musicality. This communication can either flow harmoniously or disharmoniously, depending on how the body is treated.

It is unfortunate that we often treat our bodies with less grace than the objects around us. We tend to place more value on external objects and take better care of them, neglecting the wonderful machine that is our own body. This strange phenomenon can be attributed to the egoic stories that society has ingrained in us. These fictional narratives dictate how we should look, live, treat ourselves, treat others, and even how we should feel.

It seems that mankind has deemed our bodies as not good enough. We consume external materials and alter them to fit our own preferences, believing that we know better than nature itself. We insert, eat, use, abuse, and manipulate these materials until they are unrecognisable from their natural form. And by "we," I mean our bodies.

However, let us consider what science has to say about the mechanics of the human body. Mankind may perceive the homeostasis of the body as complex, and this appears to be the only humble acknowledgment of our inability to create a human being from nothing. Instead, we were given the tools to bring life into existence. Yet, we cannot truly create a human or even an apple without utilising the tools that have already been provided for us.

Unfortunately, these facts may have been overshadowed by the egoic stories that dominate our thoughts and by those who believe themselves superior to the force that created the planet.

The Gut: The Body's Second Brain

The gut, often referred to as the second brain, serves as the body's largest messenger system. Its primary role is to maintain homeostasis, ensuring a balance in our internal chemical and physical conditions. Both the endocrine system and the nervous system play crucial roles in stimulating the gut and regulating metabolism to maintain this balance.

The endocrine system synthesises and releases over 20 different hormones to support this process. These hormones are evenly distributed across the epithelium of the gastrointestinal tract. This state of optimal performance for the organism encompasses various factors, including maintaining body temperature and fluid balance within specific predetermined boundaries.

What Are These Cells and What Do They Do?

- **Intestinal Epithelial Cells (IECs):** These line the surface of the intestinal epithelium, playing vital roles in food digestion, nutrient absorption, and protecting the body from microbial infections. Dysfunction in IECs can lead to disease (or "dis-ease"—a state of the body not being at ease). The development, maintenance, and function of IECs are strongly influenced by external nutrition, such as amino acids, which regulate their properties and functions.

- **Enteroendocrine Cells:** These hormone-producing cells are dispersed throughout the mucosal epithelium of the gastrointestinal tract, making them the largest endocrine tissue in the body. The endocrine system responds to mechanical and chemical stimuli, prompting these cells to secrete a variety of crucial hormones, including GLP-1, GLP-2, PYY, CCK, and serotonin.

- **Dissemination of Cells:** These cells extend from the stomach to the rectum, reacting to what has been consumed by releasing gut hormones such as CCK, GLP-1, GIP, peptide YY, somatostatin, ghrelin, and serotonin. These hormones regulate food intake and insulin release (Gribble & Reimann, 2016; Psichas et al., 2015).

The role of these hormones is to maintain glucose homeostasis and the equilibrium of our electrical energy.

Validating the Body

Individuals often seek acknowledgment and validation from external sources, yet they frequently neglect to listen to and validate their own bodies—regardless of the professional titles they may hold.

Epstein-Barr Virus (EBV) attempts to undermine the immune system and deplete its resources; however, the adrenal glands work to compensate, ensuring that the body continues to function. Despite the assaults from EBV, the body operates cohesively to maintain stability while combating the virus, which primarily targets the central nervous system.

EBV was initially regarded as a beneficial virus, similar to the beneficial bacteria that help regulate our immune system and assist in eliminating waste by targeting toxins within the body. Many individuals may remain unaware of their EBV status, as it can reside dormant in the body for a lifetime.

The introduction of new, toxic foods into our diets has altered the behaviour of EBV. These toxins not only pose risks to our health but also adversely affect EBV. When EBV ingests these toxins, it secretes them, thereby increasing their toxicity. In response, EBV has had to adapt for its own protection and has become more resilient.

Further developments in the 19th and 20th centuries led to the increased use of pesticides, copper, lead, petroleum, mould, and various antibiotics and medications. The prevalence of pesticides in food contributed to the emergence of glandular fever, which began to spread as a result of the toxins consumed and scavenged by EBV. Consequently, EBV transformed from a friend into an adversary. The repercussions of this shift took time to manifest, with the first case of iodine deficiency, known as Hashimoto's thyroiditis, reported in 1912 by Japanese physician Hakaru Hashimoto.

However, EBV was not identified as the underlying cause; instead, the illness was attributed to environmental factors and genetics.

This situation escalated to epidemic proportions, as thousands of women sought answers from their doctors. Unfortunately, the responses were often inadequate, with the common refrain being, "It's all in your head."

Societal norms dictate that most individuals are rarely asked about their experiences. Instead, they are gaslighted and told what their conditions are. An air of arrogance prevails—if a satisfactory answer cannot be provided, the individual is deemed to be the problem.

Leading to symptoms of:

- Hot flashes
- Fatigue
- Hair loss
- Brain fog
- Numbness in hands and feet
- Swelling
- Trouble sleeping
- Bad dreams

- Dry skin

- Skin rash

- Depression

- Aches and pain

- Heart palpitations

The best food to eat is organic, and some unwashed produce can help heal the gut because it contains elevated biotics. In contrast, fruit and vegetables treated with pesticides and waxes will not provide the same benefits.

The Healers.

Professor Arnold Ehret was born on 9 July 1866. He believed that pus- and mucus-forming foods are unnatural to eat and that a diet of fruit and vegetables, especially leafy greens, is the most healing for humans. Mucus refers to slime, mould, snot, etc.

Professor Ehret himself was discharged from the military due to heart trouble, Bright's disease, and inflammation of the kidneys. He was pronounced incurable by 21 of Europe's leading doctors.

He explored fasting and a raw food diet, which ultimately healed his body. Ehret claimed that eating natural food from nature provided the body with the nutrients it needs to heal itself. He also believed that committing cannibalism—meaning eating animals—was detrimental to human health.

Expanding on his discoveries, Ehret went on to open a clinic in Switzerland that became highly popular. He treated and cured thousands of patients who were considered incurable by medical authorities. He became one of the most prominent healthcare lecturers in Europe, saving the lives of many.

Unfortunately, Professor Ehret died after delivering a lecture on 9 October 1922. He was found dead in the street after completing four lectures on the great cure and sustaining great health. His death raised suspicions, as he had suffered a fatal blow to the back of his head. While it was officially concluded that he had fallen due to a wet pavement, some believed his work posed a threat to the meat and medical industries.

More recently, Professor Spira has studied Ehret's work and dedicated himself to the theories of the mucusless diet and its practices. Spira also believes that medication is never fully eliminated from the body but is stored for long periods, alongside man-made chemical products referred to as "food."

The belief is that all disease is a result of mucus accumulation from mucus-forming foods, which can remain in the body for decades, particularly within the digestive tract. Spira reported that the average person carries as much as 10 pounds of uneliminated faeces in their bowel from childhood, continuously accumulating as they consume mucus-forming foods. This leads to poisoning of the bloodstream and the entire system with unnatural food substances.

Disease – Its Origins

The etymology of the word "disease" originates from the 14th century, meaning discomfort or inconvenience, derived from the Old French term *desaise*, which translates to lack, want, sickness, distress, or trouble. "Dis" means "without" or "a way," and "ease" refers to comfort or relief.

Based on the research and findings of Ehret and Spira, the outcome suggests that a mucusless diet consisting of raw, non-starchy vegetables and fruits can cure all diseases of the mind and body. This indicates that true healing follows the natural medical path established by our creator, rather than the errors of man driven by egoic thinking and financial gain.

Ehret, and now Spira, aim to present the truth while respecting individuals' autonomy and free will to choose how they wish to treat their bodies. Their teachings encourage self-exploration, personal responsibility, and the freedom to make informed decisions instead of blindly following societal norms or those who disregard historical facts. Everything we need for health has already been provided on this planet, yet we continue to alter what was given to us. When we observe the state of the world, it is evident that we are becoming sicker.

Ehret stated that health cannot be bought in a bottle. His system involves cleansing the body through fasting, juicing, and following a mucusless diet. These principles are detailed in his book, *The Mucusless Diet Healing System.*

Dr Sebi

Dr Sebi, born Alfredo Bowman in Tegucigalpa, Honduras, in 1933, had no formal Western education. He moved to the United States seeking treatment for his health problems, including diabetes, asthma, and obesity. However, modern medicine could only offer medication rather than a cure.

Determined to find healing, Dr Sebi sought alternative remedies and met an herbalist in Mexico. The herbalist asked him if he believed in God, to which Dr Sebi replied, "Of course I do." The herbalist then advised him to "deliver himself to God," meaning he should only eat the foods that God created.

This led Dr Sebi to eliminate all foods deemed "good" by modern society, including animal products and processed foods. He aligned with Professor Ehret and Professor Spira in believing that there is only one disease—mucus and acidity are responsible for every illness.

Although Dr Sebi did not hold the title of "doctor" through conventional means—typically interpreted as a qualified individual who treats illness—he was regarded as a doctor by those he helped to heal. He educated people on the right foods to cure illnesses rather than merely treating symptoms with chemicals that suppress the body's natural processes.

Dr Sebi taught that processed food is largely "dead" food, preserved with chemicals to prevent rotting, much like how dead animals are treated. While these chemicals may enhance taste, this is primarily because people have been conditioned to believe they taste good. Dr Sebi explained that once he stopped eating processed foods and switched to plant-based, natural foods, he could taste the chemicals in conventionally grown vegetables, making them seem stale.

The Effects of Processed Food

Dr Sebi pointed out that when people eat processed food, they often feel hungry again within an hour or even sooner. This is because their cells have not received the nutrients they require. Instead of listening to their bodies, people have been taught to follow the cravings induced by chemical-laden food products. As a result, they continue eating these foods, leading to excessive weight gain.

We are then told that we have forgotten the feeling of fullness due to stretching our stomach and putting on weight (again, it is our fault—we are defective). We then believe that eating vegetables will not fill us, but the fact is that they do because the cells are being given the correct nutrients that a human being needs.

The body is not only consuming mucus-forming foods that block its natural functions, but it is also deficient in the vitamins and minerals it needs to survive and maintain good health. Dr Sebi stated that our creator did not make a cow and that the cow is a hybrid. He believed we should not be eating meat or drinking the pus/fluid from a hybrid animal.

This is a polite way of saying that we are consuming a murdered, mutilated body that may or may not have been previously abused. Not only that, but Dr Sebi found that when his patients refrained from eating meat, their pain began to disappear. Some of Dr Sebi's patients shared their own testimonies about being healed through his teachings. Dr Sebi said, "You do not love you. When you love you, you love the world."

Dr Sebi wanted to inform the world that we are being poisoned and that the trickery of being guided to believe in science has resulted in us viewing it as if it were a god to be worshipped and trusted. And yet, hasn't science been responsible for cruelty and the production of harmful chemicals?

All Dr Sebi was promoting was a return to nature and a diet of herbs and vegetables—food that our creator made and intended for us to eat. However, if we all followed this path, those who create chemicals would not be able to use our bodies as commodities for profit. One of the biggest relationships we have in the UK is with the NHS, and for many, this relationship lasts from birth to death. Dr Sebi stated, "Everyone has been taught to accept Western medicine and reject anything outside of that realm."

He had been fighting the pharmaceutical industry for many years, which led to powerful opposition. Dr Sebi's beliefs were in alignment with Professors Ehret and Spira, along with the herbalist from Mexico, that mucus is the root cause of all diseases in the human body. He argued that a way to heal the body is to live on an alkaline diet that balances the body's pH (potential of Hydrogen) levels. Dr Sebi was considered a threat to the FDA, AMA (American Medical Association), and the medical industry, which has instructed us on how to manage disease but never truly informed us of what disease actually is.

Dr Sebi's Legal Battle

In 1988, Dr Sebi was taken to court. The headlines read:

"Herbalist Found Not Guilty in 'Fake' Healing Case"

By HAROLD L. JAMISON

In a historic decision in Brooklyn Supreme Court on Monday, a jury of six men and six women found Alfredo Bowman not guilty on two counts of practising medicine without a licence.

Bowman, affectionately known as Dr Sebi, director of the USHA Herbal Research Institute, 616 Pacific St., Brooklyn, was arrested on 10 February 1987 by Attorney General Robert Abrams' office because of advertisements placed in the Village Voice and the Amsterdam News, which claimed a cure for AIDS.

Dr Sebi stated that he was asked to bring nine people to court with him as evidence of his claims, but instead, he brought 70 individuals whom he had cured. He won the case and later funded a treatment centre, attracting people from all over the world who sought his expertise.

Dr Sebi's Perspective on Disease

Dr Sebi posed the question of what constitutes disease, suggesting that it is often perceived as compartmentalised or individualised. For instance, one might view diabetes as distinct from leukaemia or consider sickle cell anaemia to be fundamentally different from leukaemia due to their unique characteristics.

However, Dr Sebi contended that these conditions are not inherently different; rather, they all stem from a common origin. He asserted that the mucus membrane within our biological framework becomes compromised, and the specific location of this compromise dictates the manifestation of the disease. For example:

- A breach in the mucus membrane in the nasal passages results in sinusitis.

- A similar compromise in the bronchial tubes leads to bronchitis or pneumonia in the lungs.

- Diabetes arises from issues in the pancreas.

- Conditions such as schizophrenia, paranoia, Parkinson's disease, and even insomnia are linked to disturbances in the brain.

Dr Sebi believed that the alkaline state of the gut has a significant impact on the central nervous system and the brain, influencing visual perception. He argued that the images we perceive are processed by the brain through the eyes, which serve as lenses through which we view the world. An overly acidic body creates an environment conducive to inflammation and mucus production.

Healing Through Natural Foods

To address these health issues, Dr Sebi used herbs and educated his patients about natural foods. He observed that indigenous populations, who rely on herbal medicine, tend to maintain good health without a dependency on long-term medication. He identified **glucose** as a significant enemy and recommended its avoidance.

Dr Aris, the pioneer of sun-fired food, corroborated this perspective by sharing that he has remained healthy for over 50 years by abstaining from meat and artificial products. He noted that many of the foods consumed today, including certain fruits, salads, and plant-based items, have been altered by scientific processes. Dr Aris personally concluded that "modern food has been weaponised," and he now exclusively consumes natural foods that are sun-baked.

Dr Sebi emphasised the importance of self-love by advocating for the careful selection of what one consumes, both for oneself and others. He believed that every item ingested should enhance well-being and support the nervous system. Failing to do so, he warned, may lead to discomfort, stress, and a negative self-perception.

A Legacy of Healing

Dr Sebi sought not merely to alleviate symptoms but to identify and address their **underlying causes**. He held the conviction that his arrest was a consequence of his commitment to truth and righteousness, drawing a parallel to the persecution faced by Jesus for similar teachings.

His teachings continue to inspire those seeking natural healing, and his message remains a powerful challenge to the conventional medical industry.

Dr Sebi's Teachings on Natural Healing

Dr Sebi believed that once people woke up to the realisation that natural remedies could heal their bodies, they would begin to seek them out. This, he argued, was self-empowerment.

Dr Sebi always questioned what he was told and searched for his own answers. However, this is something many of us fail to do—we have been programmed to be reliant on our puppet masters and their directives. It seems the only thing we tend to seek is *good enough* wealth and material objects, falsely believing they will bring us happiness.

Dr Sebi did not want his patients to be dependent on him. Instead, he encouraged them to love themselves, follow nature, and consume the food that nature offers—not the chemicals that man provides.

When Dr Sebi began helping people, he told his mother that he had discovered cures for several life-threatening diseases, including cancer and AIDS, and had the evidence to prove it. He recalled his mother's response: *"They are going to get you."* Dr Sebi later died in prison, having refused to eat the food he believed to be poisoned.

The Connection Between the Brain and the Body

If you eat processed food, consume the flesh of mutated animals (stressed and pumped with chemicals), drink the pus from an animal, or take pharmaceutical medication, your gut will react in much the same way as your brain does to an abnormality.

The brain speaks through mood, and the body speaks through hormones—chemical messaging through the limbic system. Just because we have been told something does not make it true, even when it is presented under the name of science.

More recently, Dr Chris Van Tulleken (2024) has spoken on multiple platforms, warning us about how ultra-processed foods are making us sick. Dr Van Tulleken states that 20% of people in the UK are getting 80% of their calories from ultra-processed food. He also informs us that this food is deliberately engineered to make us addicted to it. When examining food labels, you can clearly see the saturation of chemicals in these products.

Dr Van Tulleken has written a series of books on ultra-processed food. He was particularly disturbed when he took a trip to Brazil and witnessed the marketing strategies used by Nestlé in the Amazon. He discovered that children under the age of 10, who were consuming these products, were already suffering from Type 2 diabetes.

While Dr Van Tulleken referred to processed food as *food*, he was corrected by his Brazilian colleague, who stated:

"It is not food. It is an industrially produced edible substance."

However, *edible* implies *safe to eat*—so are these substances truly safe to consume?

The Reality of Food Processing

Nestlé S.A. is a Swiss multinational food and drink processing conglomerate, headquartered in Vevey, Switzerland. Since 2014, it has been the largest publicly held food company in the world, measured by revenue and other metrics.

The definition of *processing* is:

"To perform a series of mechanical or chemical operations on something in order to change or preserve it."

If we consume chemicals, we are blamed for eating too much of them and making ourselves sick. We are often conditioned to see ourselves as defective—because that is what we have been taught. However, when you eat natural food, you can eat as much as you like, and your body will maintain its natural size.

The Medical Industry and Its Doctrine

Medicine, as we know it, follows a doctrine that does not treat ill patients with Mother Nature's remedies but instead with synthetic chemicals. The reality is simple: you cannot make money from what has been given to us for free—or at least, not as much money.

Mother Nature's medicine has the power to cure illness. Chemicals, on the other hand, serve to fund and sustain the pharmaceutical industry.

Dr David J. Clark discovered research in 2010 that revealed a link between casein and bipolar disorder, as well as other brain disorders. He began treating a number of his patients who were suffering from bipolar disorder and observed astonishing improvements in their health. Dr Clark verified for himself that casein was responsible for immune activation.

Casein protein, present in milk, is responsible for its white colour and makes up about 80% of the protein content in cow's milk. Apart from milk, casein can also be found in yogurt, cheese, infant formulas, and various dietary supplements. When Dr Clark's patients removed all milk products from their diet, they found that their manic symptoms were relieved. However, the depressive symptoms remained.

Dr Clark states that casein causes neurological disorders. Despite opposition from some doctors, a child who had been suffering from seizures was found to be reacting to casein.

Although we are led to believe that animal products are superior to plants in terms of nutrition—and they are often the first to appear when searching for protein—it has long been known that the source of protein, whether from animals or plants, is significant.

There are evident adverse consequences linked to the prolonged consumption of high-protein, high-meat diets. These include bone and calcium imbalance disorders, heightened cancer risk, liver disorders, and the exacerbation of coronary artery disease.

It is often the loudest voice that is heard or the most persistent message that dominates. Repeated exposure to the same narratives on television and in the media influences our thoughts and feelings, but this does not necessarily mean they are correct. From my findings, true healers are those who offer the freedom of choice within the culture—free from brainwashing.

If you consume processed food, dairy products, or medication, this impacts your gut. Your gut, in turn, affects your overall health and is often referred to as the second brain (gut feeling). The body communicates through hormones, chemical messaging via the limbic system, and even through thoughts or cellular programming.

Everywhere we turn, we are confronted with examples of how we interact with ourselves and others. Society constantly reminds us that we are living longer, but are we?

Are we truly living a life of good health and happiness?

While some treatments may appear to be in our best interests, closer examination often reveals that they are not always aligned with our well-being. It seems that those who orchestrate these treatments have their own vested interests in mind, and we have become accustomed to accepting them without question.

I believe we are all healers—not only of ourselves but also of others. Most of us set out to help others in our work, regardless of our career or profession. However, the reason I refer to culture is that what we learn may not always be beneficial to us. The books we read to gain certification are guided by those who dictate what they want us to learn, preventing us from deviating outside their narrative.

We often believe what someone else has told us instead of investigating for ourselves. If we do deviate, we may be met with the indoctrination of others, or even subjected to ridicule or attack.

Case study -Cancer Cure.

This case highlights the contrast between indoctrination and human beings simply asking fellow human beings for help.

An infant named Christen lived with her family in San Francisco, where her father, Sergeant (Sgt) Schiff, worked as a police officer. Unfortunately, Christen was diagnosed with brain cancer, and the medical professionals treating her informed Sgt Schiff and his wife that, without treatment, Christen's condition would be fatal.

The proposed treatment involved extensive sessions of radiation and chemotherapy, which proved to be both barbaric and distressing for the Schiff family as they witnessed the adverse effects on Christen. Her hair fell out, and she suffered burns on her head from the radiation. Additionally, her urine became highly toxic, necessitating the use of rubber gloves during nappy changes to prevent further harm to her delicate skin and the skin of her caregivers.

Despite enduring this gruelling treatment, Christen managed to survive for six months, but the cancer persisted. The family received the devastating news that Christen's death was imminent and began preparing for the worst.

However, the Schiffs refused to give up on their daughter's life and embarked on a journey of researching cancer and exploring alternative treatments. During their search, they stumbled upon a book written by Dr Stanislaw Burzynski, which not only impressed them with his work but also revealed successful outcomes in treating cancer patients.

Determined to try another approach, the Schiffs decided to schedule Christen for treatment with Dr Burzynski, and it turned out to be a remarkable success. Not only was the treatment more humane, but Christen also became cancer-free after 18 months. Unfortunately, the cancer resurfaced in her brain, leading her to undergo further treatment from Dr Burzynski, which once again eradicated the cancer.

Tragically, Christen ultimately succumbed to neurological necrosis caused by the radiation she had received during mainstream medical treatment. This irreversible damage resulted in the permanent death of brain tissue. An autopsy conducted on Christen revealed that she was completely cancer-free.

The Schiff family expressed their heartbreak, believing that Christen had died needlessly from a cruel form of medicine, despite having found Dr Burzynski's treatment for cancer. They believed that their daughter had lost her life because they had initially been led down the wrong path.

We are raised to believe that those with professional titles know best and have our best interests at heart, especially under the label of *healthcare*. However, I believe that everyone should take the time to look at their own body, listen to their own feelings, and ask themselves: *Am I being cared for in a way that truly helps me?* and *Is there a cure?*

A professional is simply a person who has been trained in a particular field, but we can only learn what others have been taught. If someone is trained within the confines of a limited perspective, then they too remain confined. We must look beyond that box.

Think back to what we were taught in school and compare it to what we have since learned through experience. A lot of what we were taught was not true, yet that is what we pass on to others. The biggest *A-star* many of us receive in life is shaped by phrases such as *must, should, have to, got to*, and, above all, *fear*.

One of the greatest lies we are led to believe is that we must strive to be *good enough*. This belief is often triggered by the fear of losing what we think defines our worth—whether that be a label, a car, a house, an object, or even a person. As the saying goes, *we are being led down the garden path*.

Dr Burzynski's treatment is based on his discovery that individuals with peptides in their blood and urine were free of cancer, whereas those without peptides developed the disease. His idea was that, by transferring these peptides from healthy individuals to cancer patients, he could cure the illness.

When Dr Burzynski consulted his lawyer, he discovered that this kind of treatment was not governed by the Texas Food, Drug, and Cosmetic Act.

What on earth have we learnt?

When you are treated for cancer, all your cells—good, bad, and ugly—are affected by the treatment, much like a bomb going off. After the devastation, the surviving cells attempt to repair and rebuild.

Yale Medicine (2024) reports that among the frequently encountered side effects of cancer and its treatment are pain, fatigue, anaemia, oral complications, nausea, changes in weight and dietary concerns, as well as issues related to hair, skin, and nails. Pain encompasses a wide range of symptoms and is a prevalent experience across all types of cancer and their respective treatments.

Additionally, here are some other side effects you may also suffer from:

- Urinary issues
- Sleep disturbances and insomnia
- Bone density loss
- Heart damage

- Fertility issues

- Sexual health issues

- Nerve problems

- Memory or concentration problems, or delirium

- Lymphedema (lymphatic system blockage)

- Bleeding and bruising

- Edema (swelling)

Many individuals have greatly benefited from Dr Burzynski's cancer treatment. One such case is Laura. Laura was diagnosed with cancer and was undergoing the same treatment as Christen, which had been unsuccessful. She and her family asked their NHS oncologist if he would monitor her—such as by conducting blood tests—when she returned to the UK after receiving treatment at Dr Burzynski's clinic in America.

Ben Hymas, Laura's partner, recorded a call with the NHS oncologist in 2011. Ben and his family stated that, on the recording, the oncologist admitted that he did not understand Dr Burzynski. The oncologist went on to say that it was not just Dr Burzynski himself but his *Antineoplastons* approach that remained highly controversial.

Laura's family, including Ben and her parents, explained to the oncologist that Dr Burzynski was FDA-approved and that his results were extraordinary. Ben argued that Burzynski was offering something the NHS did not provide. However, the oncologist stated that monitoring Laura while she underwent this treatment was not something he could offer.

Laura's family countered with the case of a seven-year-old child who had received Dr Burzynski's treatment after being given just three months to live by an NHS oncologist. Not only was the child cured by Dr Burzynski, but the NHS doctor had agreed to monitor her, and she was now 11 years old. Ben pointed out the inconsistency in NHS policy.

The oncologist responded, *"I personally have a problem with Dr Burzynski and his individual care plan."* He ended the call by stating that, *"in my personal opinion, it will not work."* The family's trust in the NHS staff was shattered, as it seemed irresponsible to gamble with someone's life based purely on personal opinions.

Determined to proceed, the family began a fundraiser for Laura's treatment and was shocked when they received full support from actor and comedian Rufus Hound.

In 1989, Julian Whitaker, MD, expressed interest in Dr Burzynski's research. Similarly, the National Cancer Institute obtained testimonies from patients stating that Dr Burzynski's innovative treatment had successfully cured numerous individuals who had been deemed untreatable by conventional oncologists.

Kurume University Hospital, situated in Fukuoka Prefecture, Japan, began a study focused on *Antineoplastons*. The objective was to assess the effects of the treatment through direct observation. In the preliminary phase of the trial, which involved 43 participants, the safety of both oral administration and injection was confirmed.

Significantly, half of the patients involved were completely independent of Dr Burzynski and his organisation, underscoring the integrity of the research methodology employed. The results revealed that these patients experienced favourable outcomes and voiced their support for Dr Burzynski's work, thereby validating its credibility.

Unfortunately, Kurume University later announced its inability to proceed with the clinical trials required for Antineoplastons to gain market approval exclusively for the Japanese demographic. This decision was attributed to the influence of the United States FDA on the global market.

It is believed that the FDA would retaliate against any Japanese pharmaceutical company seeking approval for Antineoplastons in Japan by revoking approval for their other products in the United States. Dr Hideaki Tsuda has reported that Dr Burzynski has faced multiple legal challenges from the FDA.

Supporters among his patients have attended court proceedings, emphasising the significance of Dr Burzynski's treatment. Although the FDA has lost these cases, they have persisted in their actions, using taxpayer funds, even after the court urged them to cease their pursuit of Dr Burzynski. Many patients have expressed their long-standing struggle against the FDA.

Dr Burzynski has spoken out about the unnecessary suffering and deaths of patients due to what he describes as barbaric treatments. His dedication to assisting and curing his patients is evident, as he has financed his own research through loans, patient fees, and insurance payments.

Dr Harold Gardener remarked that, in the realm of investigative science, Dr Burzynski's research has been conducted with professionalism and is as remarkable as any other studies conducted in the state of Michigan or those with which Dr Gardener is directly associated.

He further noted that a significant portion of the health and medical industry operates as a closed system—if one proposes ideas that could potentially threaten its economic foundation, they quickly find themselves at a disadvantage. Dr Gardener has worked with several patients who opted for Dr Burzynski's treatment.

However, the availability of these treatments remains limited due to economic and organisational factors rather than scientific ones.

A campaign to sway public opinion saw patients being approached by the Honourable Texas State Board of Medical Examiners, utilising taxpayer funds to solicit complaints against Dr Burzynski. After this strategy proved unsuccessful, the medical examiners attempted to persuade Dr Burzynski to cease his patient care, leading to further investigations. Dr Burzynski provided twice the amount of evidence demonstrating that he was indeed successfully treating cancer patients.

Despite receiving this evidence, the medical examiners remained resolute. Two years later, they accused Dr Burzynski of violating a law that had been fabricated and did not exist, in yet another effort to impede his patient care. Once again, the medical board lacked a substantial case.

However, they continued their campaign against him for five years, during which patients petitioned the board to cease their harassment of Dr Burzynski. The board attempted to disregard the petition and sought to remove it from the record, culminating in a court case in May 1993.

Earl Corbilt, a retired Administrative Law Judge, reviewed the case and found no basis for the complaint from the medical examiners, as they lacked an expert witness. Dr Nicholas J. Patronas, Chief of the Section of Neuroradiology at the NIH Clinic – National Cancer Institute, was present during the proceedings.

He testified that he had referred five patients with significant brain tumours to Dr Burzynski, and their tumours had completely resolved. These patients, who were also present in court, displayed strong emotions during the hearing. Dr Patronas emphasised that the survival of these patients was not only remarkable but also astonishing.

Among Dr Burzynski's patients was a four-year-old boy named Paul, who was battling cancer and facing a grim prognosis due to the inability of conventional doctors to provide effective treatment. Paul's mother sought help from Dr Burzynski and addressed the state's attorney directly, expressing her concerns about the additional stress of potentially losing her son's treatment due to the medical examiners' actions.

The judge provided positive remarks regarding Dr Burzynski's work, noting that Paul survived and is now in his thirties, living cancer-free. Dr Burzynski also confronted the state's attorney, asserting that he operated within the law but warned that if his ability to treat patients were hindered, the attorney could face legal consequences for contributing to patient deaths. Ultimately, Dr Burzynski prevailed in the case.

However, the Honourable Medical Examiners' Board took Dr Burzynski to the Supreme Court, despite the fact that six grand juries had acquitted him. One patient requested that the FDA refrain from interfering in their lives and infringing upon doctor-patient confidentiality. The FDA continues to pursue its objectives at the expense of human health. The situation clearly indicates a lack of regard for human life; furthermore, it suggests that taxpayers' money is being utilised against the very health of the populace.

The FDA seems to promote pharmaceuticals that are financially beneficial, implying that our well-being is sustained by chemical manufacturing facilities situated in close proximity. Our options are limited to chemically enhanced food produced by one factory, followed by medical interventions from another. We are often told that our health issues are intricate; however, this complexity appears to arise from external entities motivated by profit rather than a sincere concern for our welfare.

Rather than being inherently complicated, our health is compromised. In observing the natural world, we recognise that it operates without the concept of calories, and within this natural framework, we have strayed significantly from our true human nature, adopting externally imposed narratives. We receive instructions regarding our identities, behaviours, emotions, dietary choices, clothing, thoughts, and expressions.

This conditioning has led to the normalisation of irrationality, as we have been taught to revere material wealth under the misconception that greater accumulation will lead to increased happiness and success. This phenomenon serves as a significant mechanism of control. The objects we pursue lack intrinsic value; rather, they gain significance to our well-being through the narratives we embrace, compelling us to follow blindly, much like a donkey enticed by a carrot. The biggest relationships we spend our lives in are with the food industry and the health industry.

It is noteworthy that the bioactivity of bioactive peptides primarily originates from fruits and vegetables. However, advertisements predominantly emphasise meat—the flesh of slaughtered animals—and eggs, relegating fruits and vegetables to a secondary position.

We are eating from one chemical factory to another.

Professor Thomas Seyfried holds a position as a professor of Biology at Boston College. He published a book in 2012 that posits that cancer is fundamentally a metabolic disorder linked to mitochondrial dysfunction. In his role, he instructs on cancer metabolism and general biology, aiming to enhance public understanding of these subjects.

Recognised as an authority in the field of cancer research, he is committed to investigating the underlying causes of the disease. His research is supported through private funding, and he strives to develop treatment methods that do not involve the use of toxic substances.

Despite the investment of billions of dollars and extensive research efforts, cancer continues to claim over 1,670 lives daily. Advanced "genetic" therapies and theories, alongside aggressive treatments such as radiation, chemotherapy, and surgery, have made minimal impact in reducing the toll of this enduring battle.

Cancer has been an inherent aspect of the human experience, becoming increasingly prevalent with the arrival of Western civilisation, alongside conditions such as diabetes and cardiovascular diseases. While many carcinogens, including pollution, chemicals, and tobacco, are well-documented, our comprehensive understanding of how these agents disrupt healthy cellular function remains incomplete.

Dr Seyfried's influential work, *Cancer as a Metabolic Disease: On the Origin, Management, and Prevention of Cancer*, provides an in-depth analysis of the shortcomings of current research, particularly in the realm of genetics. It emphasises how fundamental cellular biology can shed light on both the origins and potential treatments of cancer.

Dr Seyfried's hypothesis regarding impaired cellular respiration, which revisits the "Warburg Theory," presents a coherent explanation and uncovers an unexpected link to diet. This theory suggests that cancer cells lose their capacity to generate energy through oxygen utilisation and instead depend on fermentation processes. Consequently, cancer cells predominantly rely on glucose for energy, and dietary modifications that significantly lower carbohydrate consumption can effectively "starve" these cells.

Addressing the root cause rather than merely alleviating symptoms is essential. In a recent presentation, Dr Seyfried posed a question highlighting his belief that genetic markers for cancer provide more information about the effects of the disease rather than its underlying causes.

Upon examining cancer cells, Dr Seyfried observed that the mitochondria were irreversibly compromised. The absence of normal mitochondria indicates an inability to generate energy through the standard oxidative phosphorylation process. This oxidative phosphorylation is irreparably damaged in all types of cancer, irrespective of their origin, compelling the cells to rely on a fermentation mechanism. Fermentation of glutamine, sugars, and amino acids is essential; without these, cancer cells cannot survive.

Dr Seyfried discusses various factors associated with the onset of different types of cancer. For instance, breast cancer may be linked to milk consumption, colon cancer to viral infections, and lifestyle choices such as smoking, drinking, exposure to radiation, and inflammation. He posits that these detrimental influences can harm the mitochondria, resulting in abnormal cell growth or dysregulation. The behaviour of these cancerous cells resembles that of ancient cells, which thrived in an oxygen-deprived environment, relying on fermentation for energy.

Dr Seyfried argues that certain medical treatments inadvertently support the growth of cancer cells, asserting that the prevailing standard of care is illogical. For instance, therapies like radiation and temozolomide release significant amounts of glucose and glutamine within the tumour microenvironment, making long-term survival from cancer exceedingly rare. He strongly implies that such treatments may ultimately contribute to the patient's demise, particularly when radiation is applied to the brain, which he considers nonsensical.

Industrially produced vegetables are accumulating toxic species due to an unsuitable diet and a deficiency of nutritious varieties. Over 100 carcinogens can accumulate in Brussels sprouts or mushrooms, indicating that these plants employ defensive chemicals to deter predation or co-predation. Consequently, when consumed, these substances may accumulate and lead to toxic effects within our bodies, particularly due to harmful fertilisers that directly affect the mitochondria. In contrast, consuming organic produce and utilising natural fertilisers may mitigate these risks. Nevertheless, do we truly have certainty regarding the organic nature of the food we consume?

Dr Seyfried asserts that cancer hospitals continue to provide patients with sugary products. During my own visit to a hospital, I observed a menu filled with unhealthy carbohydrates and sugary beverages, with no options for organic whole foods. Furthermore, many staff members appeared to be in poor health. This observation can be disconcerting when one enters a healthcare facility and notices that many individuals responsible for providing care do not prioritise their own well-being.

This situation may be interpreted as a form of wilful ignorance. I have often heard medical professionals assert, "We do not understand why the body functions in certain ways" or "It is simply one of those things." Such remarks seem to lack scientific depth. Should our tax contributions not warrant a more thorough exploration? There is a steady influx of funding directed towards cancer research, despite the prevalence of initiatives such as coffee mornings featuring baked goods. This is particularly noteworthy, as the very items offered at these gatherings are recognised as detrimental to health.

Does this not represent a superficiality that conceals the evident truth?

We consume foods laden with chemicals and are then treated with additional chemical medications. The presence of chemical manufacturing plants appears to flourish, yet the overall health of the population continues to deteriorate.

The conclusions drawn by Dr Seyfried are consistent with Dr Burzynski's claim that this type of treatment is inhumane and should be halted. Dr Sebi stated, "Due to man's biology, we are of the organic family. We need to change our diet to that which is compatible with our cellular predisposition."

He went on to state, "Chemotherapy is an approach that destroys cells—whether they are good cells or bad cells, they get destroyed. It is an acid approach." Dr Sebi's approach focused on intracellular cleansing by identifying the root cause of disease and removing it.

There has been a lack of meaningful advancement in these therapies for almost a century. But this makes sense—how can you patent nature? However, you can patent chemicals, and if nature makes you well, then there is no business model.

Dr Seyfried raises concerns about the justification for administering drugs that are often feared by cancer patients due to their severe side effects, especially when there are less invasive options available, such as eliminating harmful fuels and adopting non-toxic therapeutic ketosis. He noted that it is impossible for individuals to benefit from appropriate treatment methods, as patients are often not presented with this choice. Some promising drug therapies are considered inappropriate despite their potential in cancer treatment, particularly when used in conjunction with nutritional therapeutic ketosis.

Likewise, Dr Burzynski and Dr Sebi have encountered considerable criticism for their perspectives. Dr Seyfried acknowledges that numerous oncologists are hesitant to recognise the efficacy of alternative therapies, frequently citing a lack of supporting evidence. Nevertheless, they appear to overlook the considerable evidence highlighting the detrimental effects of their own treatments, which have been deemed inhumane.

The Original Oath

It was written:

Hippocratic Oath (ca. 400 bce)

Translated by Francis Adams.

http://classics.mit.edu/Hippocrates/hippooath.html.

"I SWEAR by Apollo the physician, and Aesculapius, and Health, and Allheal, and all the gods and goddesses, that, according to my ability and judgment, I will keep this Oath and this stipulation-to reckon him who taught me this Art equally dear to me as my parents, to share my substance with him, and relieve his necessities if required; to look upon his offspring in the same footing as my own brothers, and to teach them this art, if they shall wish to learn it, without fee or stipulation; and that by precept, lecture, and every other mode of instruction, I will impart a knowledge of the Art to my own sons, and those of my teachers, and to disciples bound by a stipulation and oath according to the law of medicine, but to none others. I will follow that system of regimen which, according to my ability and judgment, I consider for the benefit of my patients, and abstain from whatever is deleterious and mischievous.

I will give no deadly medicine to any one if asked, nor suggest any such counsel; and in like manner I will not give to a woman a pessary to produce abortion. With purity and with holiness I will pass my life and practice my Art. I will not cut persons laboring under the stone, but will leave this to be done by men who are practitioners of this work. Into whatever houses I enter, I will go into them for the benefit of the sick, and will abstain from every voluntary act of mischief and corruption; and, further from the seduction of females or males, of freemen and slaves.

Whatever, in connection with my professional practice or not, in connection with it, I see or hear, in the life of men, which ought not to be spoken of abroad, I will not divulge, as reckoning that all such should be kept secret.

While I continue to keep this Oath unviolated, may it be granted to me to enjoy life and the practice of the art, respected by all men, in all times! But should I trespass and violate this Oath, may the reverse be my lot!"

Hippocrates was recognised by the followers of Pythagoras for connecting medicine and philosophy. He separated religion from medicine, challenging the false belief that disease was a punishment from the gods. Instead, Hippocrates argued that disease stemmed from a person's diet, living habits, and environmental factors.

Despite this oath being written over 2,500 years ago, there appears to be a new belief. Instead of divine punishment, it now seems that the fault lies in the very creation of human beings. Once again, we are rendered powerless when told that our DNA is faulty and serves as the marker for our illness and disease—implying that our fate is sealed.

However, it may be that our genes are activated due to an environment filled with toxins and chemicals, both in the air and in the food we consume. When the microbiome is in a healthy state, it communicates this balance. Conversely, if the microbiome becomes disturbed—such as from excessive protein intake—protein fermenters break down the protein, producing ammonia. This can lead to a build-up of mucus, resulting in conditions like pneumonia. In such cases, the microbiome signals its distress, as it is merely trying to survive.

We are often medicated for the symptoms but are not informed of the underlying causes or how to prevent adverse reactions to the chemicals we consume.

The Chemical Doctors

There is a Hippocratic Oath in the DSM-5 that upholds the approach of "Do No Harm," which doctors sign. The original version of the Hippocratic Oath states:

"I will use my power to help the sick to the best of my ability and judgement. I will abstain from harming or wronging man by it."

These words have been set as a guideline. However, I cannot see how this can be a guideline if an oath is deemed a promise—a declaration or assurance that one will do something.

I understand that we may not always realise when we offend others or hurt their feelings, and it may not be our intention. However, I struggle to see how this oath can truly apply in medicine. The wording itself is absolute—"DO NO HARM"—not "do a little bit of harm," but "do no harm," even if it is framed as a guideline.

How can a doctor sign such an oath while training and knowingly entering a profession that dispenses chemicals—medications—without fully understanding their long-term effects on the human body? I have never seen a medication that has no side effects, meaning some degree of harm is always done to the body. Many in the medical profession justify this by saying, "If the benefits outweigh the risks."

But what is the meaning of risk?

"Risk is the likelihood that a person may be harmed or suffer adverse health effects if exposed to a hazard."

Furthermore, in my experience, challenging this notion can often be met with anger, verbal abuse, gaslighting, arguments, or even silence. I am not saying there is no kindness in medicine, nor am I saying that healthcare professionals do not intend to do good. However, ignorance is a choice—especially when substantial evidence points to systemic problems.

According to Fieldfisher:

"In law, duty of care is defined as a duty to provide care at a level reasonably expected of any competent doctor, nurse, midwife, surgeon, etc. A newly qualified GP, for example, would be expected to provide the same level of safe care as someone more experienced when performing the same task."

The *Journal of the American Medical Association* (2010) and *The British Medical Journal* (2016) both agree that the three biggest killers are:

1. Cardiovascular disease

2. Cancer

3. Iatrogenic causes (from the Greek *iatrogenic*, meaning a state of ill health or adverse effects caused by medical treatment)

Recent research suggests that medical errors could be responsible for up to 251,000 deaths each year in the United States, making them the third leading cause of death. The rate of medical errors in the U.S. is significantly higher compared to other developed nations like Canada, Australia, New Zealand, Germany, and the United Kingdom.

Shockingly, fewer than 10 per cent of medical errors are officially documented. One study evaluated the effectiveness of the MEDMARX Medication Error Reporting system across 25 hospitals in Pennsylvania. The data analysed included 17,000 errors reported by these hospitals within a 12-month timeframe.

In the UK, the NHS is responsible for hundreds of millions of prescribing errors and mix-ups annually, leading to an estimated 22,300 deaths each year, according to a major government-commissioned report. Mistakes range from inadequate monitoring of patients on potent medications and poor communication between GPs and hospitals to administering the wrong drugs altogether.

The risks associated with these errors vary from minor incidents—such as providing the wrong strength of an inhaler—to life-threatening mistakes, such as mixing up medications for critically ill patients.

Prescription medications are now the third leading cause of death in the United States and Europe, following heart disease and cancer. Of those who die, approximately half adhered to their medication regimen, while the other half succumbed to errors—such as incorrect dosages or being prescribed drugs with contraindications.

Regulatory agencies provide little assistance in preventing these deaths, relying on superficial solutions like lengthy warning lists, precautions, and contraindications for each medication. However, it is unrealistic to expect doctors to memorise every single risk.

The prevalence of drug-related fatalities can be linked to ineffective drug regulation, widespread corruption (such as falsified scientific data and bribery of healthcare professionals), and deceptive marketing strategies that are as harmful as historical tobacco advertising—and should be banned in the same way.

To protect themselves, patients should minimise their reliance on medications, carefully read package inserts, and consult reputable sources like Cochrane Reviews to make informed choices. People should feel empowered to reject medications when necessary.

What is also revealing is how we have been conditioned to seek medical intervention whenever we feel unwell. The first response to illness is often, *"Have you been to the doctor?"* or *"You should go to the doctor."*

Another striking observation is that research phrases medical errors as "causes of death" rather than attributing responsibility to individuals or institutions. Why is this? Does it remove accountability? If someone's death results from medical negligence or improper prescription, should it not be considered manslaughter—or even murder?

Even if unintentional, prescribing chemicals that cause harm while accepting the doctrine of *"if the benefits outweigh the risks"* raises ethical concerns. When will a collective awakening occur? When will we truly acknowledge that the estimated 22,300 lives lost each year—people seeking help—represent a catastrophic failure?

This brings us to the concept of *wilful blindness*. In medicine, professionals are taught to report anyone who poses a risk to themselves or others. Yet, we turn a blind eye to the inherent risks within the medical system itself.

Health and wellbeing are gifts from our Creator, and yet, we take risks with our lives by placing blind trust in individuals wearing professional labels—individuals working within a system that, despite good intentions, continues to operate with dangerous flaws.

Germ Theory

Louis Pasteur is widely acknowledged as the pioneer of modern immunology due to his research in the late 19th century, which promoted the germ theory of disease. His work also introduced the idea that prophylactic vaccination could prevent all infectious diseases and that therapeutic vaccination could treat them if administered promptly after infection.

Despite working during a time when the concept of the immune system was not fully understood, Pasteur recognised how it defends against microbial invasion. His insights were ground-breaking, especially considering that distinctions between fungi, bacteria, and viruses had not yet been established, and theories of immunity had not been formulated.

Although Pasteur's understanding of immunity was flawed—he initially believed that attenuated microbes depleted essential nutrients in the host rather than triggering an active immune response—his focus on immunity laid the foundation for future advancements in the field.

However, he later refuted this theory and aligned with Bernard, who argued that disease arises from the condition of the body due to both internal and external environmental factors.

The problem with Pasteur's beliefs is that they were laden with flaws, and subsequent advancements followed a path that moved further away from understanding the human body holistically. While vaccinations may appear to eliminate some infections, at what cost to the human body? It is ultimately the body that bears the burden of repairing the damage caused by a vaccine.

For example, Dr David Campbell reports in a viral vaccine study:

"Report: 1 in 20 people had an adverse effect from the early vaccines given in the 2021 batch EJ6134. Then, in batch EW6126, 1 in 1,000 had an adverse effect. The data from the following batch is not yet available at the time of this paper."

The germ theory created a belief that we are not responsible for our own bodies and that they are inherently inefficient without chemical intervention. Removing individual responsibility allows those who oversee our food supply and medical treatments to govern us with theories that may not be true. In fact, there is a great deal of information that people believe to be true, when in reality, it may not be.

One such belief is that human intelligence has increased as we evolve. But is this actually true?

Rather than becoming more intelligent, we have become more controlled and disconnected from our true nature. Not only have humans become physically and psychologically sicker, but we have also become so entrenched in certain beliefs that it is difficult to break free from the doctrine we have been programmed with since birth.

The human body possesses an inherent ability to heal itself. From the moment we are born, we are conditioned to believe that external aids—such as bandages—are necessary for recovery when we sustain injuries. In reality, it is our body that performs the healing process.

This conditioning instils a fear of germs within us. For instance, when we suffer a fracture, a cast is applied to stabilise the limb; however, it is ultimately the body's own mechanisms that facilitate bone healing. This illustrates that, given the appropriate conditions and environment, the human body is fully capable of self-repair.

This phenomenon is also evident in the harsh treatments for cancer, which often indiscriminately destroy both healthy and malignant cells. Consequently, the body is compelled to engage in a reparative process to mend the damage inflicted by radiation and chemotherapy, highlighting the body's resilience in the face of such interventions.

The environment inside and outside of the body should be in line with our blueprint. Our cells hold the blueprint to renew themselves, meaning we are designed to function in harmony with the food we eat.

A ribosome is a cellular structure composed of RNA and protein, serving as the site for protein synthesis within the cell. It reads the messenger RNA (mRNA) sequence and converts the genetic information into a specific sequence of amino acids, which ultimately form proteins. The ribosome is a vital component responsible for protein production within cells. Comprised of two subunits, it attaches to the mRNA and moves along the molecule, decoding each three-letter codon. Acting as a binding site for tRNA, the ribosome ensures that the correct amino acids are added to the growing protein chain. Once the protein is complete, the ribosome disassembles.

For a healthy internal environment, the body requires polysaccharides, amino acids, and minerals:

- **Polysaccharides** are abundant natural polymers found in plants, animals, and microorganisms. They possess remarkable characteristics and perform vital functions essential for sustaining life. Renowned for their significant nutritional value, they have a beneficial impact on immune and digestive functions, as well as the body's detoxification system.

- **Amino acids** serve as crucial molecules utilised by all living organisms for protein synthesis. In order for the body to function optimally, it requires a total of 20 distinct amino acids. Among these, nine are classified as essential amino acids, meaning they must be obtained through dietary sources. These essential amino acids can be found in a diverse range of foods.

- **Minerals**, along with vitamins, are crucial nutrients required by the body. These two groups are collectively referred to as micronutrients because they are needed in smaller amounts compared to macronutrients such as carbohydrates and proteins. The body is unable to produce minerals on its own, so they must be obtained through diet. Different foods contain varying levels of vitamins, minerals, and other macronutrients, underscoring the importance of maintaining a balanced and diverse diet that encompasses all food groups.

A point to consider is that when searching for the proteins and minerals needed for the body, animal products and their by-products are often advertised first. While we have been taught that some of these proteins can be obtained from animal products, in my view, this is because animals themselves consume protein. However, just because animals eat from the same provider (the one that made the apple) does not necessarily mean they are intended to be killed by us.

We all have choices, and I respect yours. I only ask you to consider—are your choices truly your own, or are they the result of conditioning?

If you are not getting the correct minerals, the information within your blueprint becomes disrupted, leading to mutations that arise from what you consume. If your diet is deficient or contains chemicals or radiation—whether from food, personal care products such as creams, lotions, and shampoos, household cleaning products, or exposure to technological devices like mobile phones and laptops—this can impact your blueprint and, ultimately, your overall health.

.

The Microbiome and their Reaction to Chemicals

It is believed that photosynthetic bacteria, or cyanobacteria, are the most abundant life form on Earth. For several years, researchers have been attempting to 're-wire' the photosynthesis mechanisms of cyanobacteria to extract energy from them. There are over five trillion bacteria saturating the Earth, the atmosphere, and everything within it. These bacteria are the key to life itself.

Deoxyribonucleic acid (DNA) does not determine that you are destined to be the same as your ancestors before you. The microbiome communicates with our genes. We tend to eat the same foods or products as our family members and carry on the same habits, just as we do with Sunday lunch, known as a tradition.

It is the tradition of illness that we pass on, or the tradition of health, depending primarily on our food intake and the environmental programming we are exposed to.

There are over 40 trillion bacteria living in and on the human body. These bacteria are known as the microbiome. Without the human body being saturated with the microbiome, it would—and could—not exist. It is believed that the body is only 10% human, with the rest composed of microbiomes.

We have been taught to fear and kill the very thing we exist in. The central system for the microbiome is the gut, which acts as the brain for the body's functions. Thanks to the microbiome producing compounds that signal systems throughout the body, it takes care of the body's needs and maintains healthy function. It has been questioned whether it is the microbiome or the body's endocrine system that is truly in charge.

The endocrine system has been described as a complex network of organs and glands. In other words, as we cannot create a human, our knowledge of these systems is still very limited. This system is believed to control our growth, development, and reproduction, as well as affect the hypothalamus, regulate hormones, and impact mood, to name just a few functions.

The microbiome is certainly the driving force behind maintaining a healthy ecosystem within the body. However, the environment required to sustain a healthy microbiome has changed drastically throughout history. The increasing control exerted by external forces has caused mass hysteria and has had a devastating impact on the health of all species on the planet, including human beings.

The impact of a toxic environment on the human body is clear for all to see. Throughout history, our environment has changed to the point where good health is rarely spoken about.

For example, consider how the brain is constantly bombarded with mass hysteria from television, where illness has been so normalised and junk food is encouraged. Disease and poor mental health in the human body have become the new normal—accepted rather than questioned by many.

The microbiome is a key player in defending the body against illness and infection. When the gut microbiome suffers from dysbiosis—a loss of overall bacterial diversity, a reduction in beneficial bacteria, and an overgrowth of potentially pathogenic bacteria—it leads to a condition known as gut imbalance. This can also impact the thyroid and immune system, creating inflammation and affecting metabolism.

The simplest path to gut health is to eat uncomplicated food— the kind that has no label with a long list of ingredients you cannot understand because they are additives or binders. Nature flows, and we are part of that flow. If we take care of our microbiome, it will take care of us.

Our gut is like soil. If we spray pesticides or weed killer onto the soil, we destroy the life within it. That is exactly what we pour onto our microbiomes when we consume harmful substances.

We are constantly told to save the planet and protect nature, yet this message seems contradictory because we are nature itself. We have been led away from our humanness and the natural world for the sake of profit, damaging the ecosystem both inside our bodies and externally.

Profit has nothing to do with nature—nature takes care of itself when left undisturbed. After all, it managed to exist before we arrived.

Isabell Thomas

Changing Nature.

10,000 years ago, humans saw grass as food. The wild grass that was eaten is believed to have contained 14 chromosomes, compared to the wheat consumed today, which contains 42 chromosomes. Human beings have 46 chromosomes.

However, in the 1960s and 1970s, some wheat varieties were developed in a laboratory. This wheat was thicker and more robust than natural wheat, with the aim of benefiting farmers. We can only presume that, for example, a wheat farmer did not intend to harm nature by using pesticides. This may be largely due to ignorance, as we often fail to see small creatures as significant in nature's ecosystem.

Our egocentric, narcissistic level of consciousness made the plant all about us and our survival. When we see or experience something that we do not like—something that irritates us or obstructs our goals—we label it as a pest and invent a pesticide to kill it, alongside modifying the wheat.

Failing to recognise that everything not man-made is part of nature, we destroy creatures deemed as pests while also consuming the pesticides ourselves. Does the benefit outweigh the risk in this case? What do these modifications and pesticides do to our microbiomes? The imbalance in nature's ecosystem exists both inside and outside of us because everything is interconnected. If you disrupt the balance externally, you disrupt the balance internally.

Wheat contains glutamine. Gluten, comprising approximately 80% of wheat protein, is a structural protein primarily composed of glutenin and gliadins. Gliadin molecules contain antigenic sites that may trigger immune activation, leading to conditions such as coeliac disease—an inflammatory condition affecting the gut. Furthermore, geneticists modified wheat to increase glycine betaine.

Although this may have been unintentional at the time, these changes altered the microbiome's response. Wheat now contains gliadin protein, which increases appetite and cravings for processed products, largely due to the sugar content in wheat-based foods such as bread, cakes, and biscuits. Wheat also contains exorphins—an addictive property.

Dr Efrat La Mandre indicates that gluten and gliadin proteins contribute to the development of Hashimoto's disease and coeliac disease. These proteins are known to compromise the integrity of the intestinal lining, leading to a condition commonly referred to as leaky gut. This issue may be further exacerbated by the various additives present in modern wheat.

Additionally, research suggests that consuming wheat can temporarily induce a heightened state of leaky gut, even in individuals without autoimmune diseases, and is associated with inflammation. Dr David J. Clarke also points out that wheat consumption may lead to symptoms such as dizziness, vertigo, and balance disturbances.

These symptoms indicate underlying inflammation, which can affect the inner ear. This phenomenon is linked to immune system messengers known as cytokines, which are present in all neurons and play a role in signal processing. An imbalance in the distribution of cytokines, particularly those responsible for relaying information from the inner ear, can alter nerve circuits.

Gluten has been observed to cross-react with various substances. This occurs when antibodies bind not solely to one target but also to another with similar molecular structures. Physicians often describe this as the immune system's attachment process. However, it is more accurately characterised as the antibody recognising a foreign entity that shares molecular similarities with the body, such as the thyroid. This concept is known as molecular mimicry or epitope mimicry. A similar reaction can occur with dairy products.

Additionally, sugar contributes to vertigo and dizziness due to its effects on insulin resistance, which leads to inflammation.

Some individuals without Hashimoto's disease or coeliac disease may still experience symptoms such as bloating, diarrhoea, headaches, or skin rashes after consuming gluten-containing foods. This reaction may be due to poorly digested carbohydrates, such as FODMAPs, which ferment in the gut. Those with sensitive digestive systems may experience discomfort from this fermentation rather than from gluten itself.

Research indicates that some individuals may have malfunctioning small intestines with a permeable lining, allowing undigested gluten, bacteria, or other substances to pass into the bloodstream, leading to inflammation.

Even after switching to a gluten-free diet, individuals who consume processed foods may still experience weight gain, blood sugar fluctuations, and other health issues. Therefore, it is not gluten itself causing these problems, but rather the sodium, sugar, and other additives present in processed foods. The body is not receiving the right nutrients, and as a result of consuming addictive chemicals, cravings for more unhealthy substances persist.

Phytates can cause issues for many individuals due to their ability to bind to minerals and block enzyme function. When the body eliminates some phytates, it also removes minerals such as magnesium, calcium, zinc, and iron, which are bound to the phytates.

Digestive issues, mineral deficiencies, bodily pain, hormone imbalances, disrupted pH balance, anxiety, neurological disorders, paranoia in children, and brain fog have all been linked to wheat consumption. Additionally, wheat has been associated with fibromyalgia and obesity.

What remains in the body are bacteria from the large bowel, which enter the small bowel, are absorbed, and travel into the bloodstream. Due to increased gut permeability, particles flow freely into the bloodstream, including toxins and other foreign substances known as antigens, waste, and lipopolysaccharides (LPS). LPS triggers the release of pro-inflammatory substances such as TNF-α, IL-6, nitric oxide, and cyclooxygenase.

Furthermore, LPS is implicated in various conditions, including neurodegenerative disorders, acute respiratory distress syndrome, vascular diseases, and periodontal diseases.

High concentrations of LPS can activate nociceptors—specialised peripheral sensory neurons that detect harmful stimuli. These neurons relay information about injury to the brain. Pain, as a complex somatic sensation, involves both cognitive and emotional responses triggered by actual or perceived tissue damage.

This can result in the manifestation of specific behavioural or psychological responses, such as anxiety, due to the increase in corticosteroid-releasing hormone. This occurs due to the disruption of communication between the hypothalamic-pituitary-adrenal (HPA) axis. Although gluten-free products are available as an alternative, these products are often processed.

A high percentage of those who have abstained from eating wheat have resolved the health problems caused by geneticists and agribusiness. Many have reported relief from conditions such as diabetes, acid reflux, asthma, rheumatoid arthritis, obesity, and endotoxaemia.

Obesity, in one sense, can mean that individuals are blamed for eating the very food they are programmed to consume. While we are responsible for taking care of ourselves, this is a trap many fall victim to. However, once we have the right information, it becomes a matter of personal choice.

We must recognise that we are brainwashed by information from so-called experts, yet our bodies always tell us the truth. The body is the one we should listen to—you know how *you* feel.

The Making of Coca-Cola

Coca-Cola has a rich history that has been extensively documented. In 1885, John Pemberton, a pharmacist from Atlanta, Georgia, created the beverage by formulating the original recipe in his backyard. The recipe included cocaine extracted from the coca leaf, which influenced the naming of the drink as *Coca*. The *Cola* part of the name was derived from the kola nut, which contains caffeine—another stimulant.

At the time of Coca-Cola's invention, cocaine was legal and widely used in medicinal products. It was believed to be safe for consumption in small quantities (National Institute of Drug Abuse).

Diet Coke is marketed as a healthier product based on its nutritional information. However, its ingredients include carbonated water and caramel E150d, which is a mixture of chemicals, including ammonia, sulphites, aspartame, and anastrozole foam.

In late 2023, aspartame made headlines due to its classification as a possible carcinogen—a substance capable of causing cancer.

Then there is phosphoric acid, a substance that leaches minerals from bones and contributes to tooth decay.

Ultra-Processed Foods (UPFs)

The ingredients in ultra-processed foods (UPFs) commonly originate from four staple crops: rice, wheat, corn, and soy. UPFs are made from the cheapest ingredients, often considered waste commodity crops, and contain:

- Refined bleached deodorised fat/oil
- Modified starches
- Protein isolates

These are then combined with additives, including:

- Stabilisers
- Flavours
- Colours
- Emulsifiers
- Taste enhancers
- Preservatives

These ingredients are often fed to animals, with humans consuming what is essentially the leftovers. Breaking these crops down into fat, carbohydrates, and proteins adds value and extends shelf life while keeping production costs low. These products can be shipped worldwide in vast quantities, and to make them palatable, they are often combined with small amounts of meat or fish—typically pork, beef, or chicken.

The key additives in UPFs are stabilisers and emulsifiers, which bind the basic ingredients together to create texture. This allows the products to be baked, fried, extruded, pressed, and shaped.

This process is used in the majority—if not all—of the packaged food found in weekly grocery shops, including pizza, bread, cakes, and other cheaply made products with little to no nutritional value. Despite this, many UPFs are misleadingly marketed as healthy, such as chewy bars, breakfast bars, or nutritional drinks. This has become the UK's staple diet.

Come to think of it, I have never seen a food product labelled as *unhealthy*. Even foods marketed as organic can be deceptive when they contain emulsifiers such as mono- and diacetyl.

This is concerning, especially for children who are at the mercy of adults to educate them and take care of their wellbeing. However, studies show that this responsibility is increasingly neglected due to wilful ignorance or blindness. Many parents fail to consider the health of their children as they continue to poison themselves.

McDonald's Fries

Ingredients: Potatoes, vegetable oil (canola oil, corn oil, soybean oil, hydrogenated soybean oil, natural beef flavour [wheat and milk derivatives]), dextrose, sodium acid pyrophosphate (to maintain colour), salt. *Natural beef flavour contains hydrolysed wheat and hydrolysed milk as starting ingredients.*

In the UK and Europe, around 2,500 additives are used in our food, which are somewhat regulated. In the United States, there are between 5,000 and 15,000 additives, yet the FDA does not appear to have a definitive list—despite being the regulatory body for food.

The Truth About Sugar

Sugar has earned a bad reputation as it is linked to a variety of diseases, including obesity, cancer, diabetes, and heart disease. However, it has also been argued that sugar is essential for both the body and life itself.

It is crucial to understand which types of sugar are beneficial and which are harmful. Sugar that does not come from a natural source, such as fruit, is often an unnatural substance.

Your body is constantly working to repair the damage inflicted upon it. Unnatural sugar is primarily produced from sugar cane or sugar beets and is refined using chemicals such as sulphur dioxide, phosphoric acid, calcium hydroxide, and activated carbon. This process strips away all the natural nutrition originally present in the sugar.

By refining sugar down to sucrose and removing its vitamins, minerals, proteins, enzymes, and other beneficial nutrients, what remains is a concentrated unnatural substance that the human body struggles to process, let alone use.

It is interesting to note that raw sugar—often assumed to be a natural form of sugar—is also refined. Once the cane juice crystals are harvested, they undergo washing, boiling, filtering, and drying. This process removes most of the fibre and nutrients that existed in the original crystals.

As a result, the sugar becomes refined with no nutritional value. The use of artificial sweeteners is often a case of trading one problem for another and is not a path to good health. In fact, artificial sweeteners are even more harmful than refined sugar.

The Dangers of Sugar Addiction

Sugar can be a deadly addiction. People not only develop a strong taste for it but also an insatiable craving. Refined sugar stresses the pancreas and depletes the body's supply of chromium. A common symptom of chromium deficiency is sugar cravings. Satisfying these cravings further reduces chromium levels, increasing the desire for more sugar.

Furthermore, refined sugar depletes the body of all B vitamins and leaches calcium from the hair, bones, blood, and teeth. As if that were not enough, sugar also affects digestion. It ferments in the gut and inhibits the secretion of gastric juices, impairing the body's ability to digest food.

The result? Weight gain, mood swings, and irritability. These side effects stem from sugar's chemical reaction in the brain, where it releases serotonin, tricking the body into experiencing a temporary high. This leads to a spike in blood glucose levels, followed by a crash that leaves you feeling tired, irritable, and even depressed.

Natural vs. Refined Sugars

Intrinsic sugars are natural sugars found in fruit and vegetables. These sugars are not harmful to your health and are not fattening, despite what some healthcare providers may claim. Natural sugars found in fruit, vegetables, and honey are unprocessed and therefore rich in fibre and nutrients.

A diet high in fruit and vegetables ensures that your body receives the small amount of sugar it needs while providing far more health benefits than refined sugar.

Pesticides

The policy of Friends of the Earth indicates that a metric similar to Cornell University's Environmental Impact Quotient (EIQ) can be employed to evaluate the relative toxicities of pesticides currently in use in the UK.

The ecological dimension of the EIQ examines the toxicity levels affecting wildlife. The average ecological component for the top 50 pesticides used in the UK is recorded at 11.7; however, some pesticides demonstrate significantly elevated toxicity levels, raising serious concerns about their ongoing application.

The fungicide chlorothalonil, for example, possesses an ecological component of 33.1, signifying a high level of toxicity. Although it is the most prevalent pesticide used in arable farming in the UK, its application has escalated from under 0.5 million kg in 2000 to more than 2 million kg by 2016. Recently, the European Union enacted a ban on this substance.

Another pesticide of significant concern is the broad-spectrum herbicide pendimethalin, which has an EIQ of 55.8. Although it was considered for replacement by the European Commission in 2015, it received re-approval in 2017, leading to increased use on cereal crops. It is crucial to prioritise the reduction of these highly toxic pesticides and others, as continued reliance on harmful chemicals will persist until they are systematically eliminated.

Since 2000, a new category of pesticides called neonicotinoids has seen a substantial rise in usage. The most prevalent neonicotinoid in 2016 was clothianidin, applied to 728,000 acres of arable crops. Clothianidin is among the three neonicotinoids that have been banned by the EU for outdoor crop use due to their adverse effects on bee species.

It is worth noting that this decision was based on sub-lethal impacts such as colony survival and queen bee production, factors not accounted for in EIQ assessments. The three prohibited neonicotinoids were primarily used as seed treatments, representing preventive strategies implemented before any pest invasion. Research indicates that only a small percentage of these systemic pesticides effectively reach the intended pest, raising concerns about their widespread application.

Like all chemicals, they do not discriminate in their effects—they are toxic to all nature. The diverse microbiome species in the soil must be protected, as they play a crucial role in maintaining the health of all living organisms, including humans. We are exposed to a cocktail of toxins. In addition, wheat, grain, and sugars are not naturally suited to the human body due to contamination.

Our gut bacteria are responsible for synthesising vitamins B and K and engage in continuous communication with one another. They possess the ability to mutate and can influence the DNA within the host's cells. When microbiomes encounter toxins that do not align with the organism's natural structure—such as processed foods, hormone-injected meats, or pesticide-treated produce—problems can arise. This includes substances like sugar, meat, dairy, and certain vegetables.

Additionally, toxins found in household cleaning products, toothpaste, deodorants, mouthwash, and gardening supplies can provoke a reaction from the microbiome, potentially leading to disease within the body. Conditions such as irritable bowel syndrome (IBS), Crohn's disease, asthma, rosacea, psoriasis, and eczema may manifest, particularly following antibiotic treatment. Other complications may include weight gain, insulin resistance, diabetes, hypothyroidism, and hyperlipidaemia—characterised by elevated lipid levels, including cholesterol and triglycerides, in the bloodstream. These factors contribute to an increased risk of coronary heart disease, metabolic syndrome, cancer, and autoimmune disorders.

The substances and chemicals added to food to prevent the spoilage of seeds and grains include natural preservatives such as sand and stone binders, as well as chemicals like pesticides, including hydrogen, which are used to prolong the shelf life of products such as cakes. Additionally, trans fats and aspartame are employed as sweeteners. Aspartame contains aspartic acid, an amino acid, and methanol, which is harmful to the brain and nervous system.

The consumption of meat, particularly processed and red varieties, increases the risk of cancer. This heightened risk is attributed to chemicals such as nitrates and sodium phosphate, which are used to maintain the appearance of freshness in carcasses. Research indicates that approximately 41 million people die annually, with 74% of global fatalities resulting from various diseases.

The gut microbiome, a community of microbes residing in our gut, can be influenced by substances ingested both orally and through the skin, including prescription medications. Certain medications, such as antibiotics, are designed to eliminate harmful bacteria and other organisms but can also impact beneficial microbes. Meanwhile, medications like corticosteroids can reduce inflammation while encouraging the growth of yeasts such as candida, leading to an imbalance in the gut microbiome.

A study examining more than 1,000 commonly prescribed non-antibiotic medications revealed that 24% of them can disrupt the growth of at least one species of bacteria in the microbiome. This means that when taking medication, there is a 24% chance that it affects the diversity and composition of your gut microbiome, with the likelihood increasing with the use of multiple medications.

The research primarily focused on non-antibiotic medications; however, several of these drugs demonstrated antibiotic-like properties by suppressing the proliferation of certain bacterial species within the microbiome. This unforeseen result also highlights the potential risk of non-antibiotic medications contributing to the development of antibiotic resistance.

Given the escalating issues surrounding antibiotic resistance, this finding is particularly concerning. Some of the most powerful treatments available for various diseases can be likened to detonating a grenade within the human body, indiscriminately eliminating all bacteria encountered.

The microbiome's reaction to what we consume can often prevent it from functioning properly, hindering its ability to process the vitamins and minerals necessary for maintaining health. Instead, an imbalanced microbiome can lead to the leakage of toxins into the body when attempting to break down substances we have ingested.

Hormonal levels are significantly affected, leading to health complications as the metabolites fail to regulate the body's oestrogen. Studies indicate that bacteria utilise a process known as quorum sensing, which occurs when they generate specific molecules. Similarly, insects exhibit a comparable form of communication when determining the optimal locations for rest that provide the greatest advantages.

The microbiome within the human body plays a crucial role in communicating with the brain. It can utilise the endocrine system to relay information, particularly when adjustments are needed in response to stress or other bodily changes. It serves as a vital source of guidance for various bodily systems, maintaining a continuous dialogue to promote overall health.

When the microbiome is content with our dietary choices, it often results in a positive emotional state, as it releases serotonin into the brain, originating from the gut. This communication occurs via the endocrine system, utilising hormones to convey messages that influence emotional well-being, stress management, and the regulation of essential bodily functions, including metabolism, growth, and reproduction.

The primary mode of communication for the immune system is through cytokines. These are messenger molecules that convey information regarding injury and inflammation to maintain bodily equilibrium. However, if the microbiome is compromised, astrocytes—cells located in the central nervous system and brain— can become excessively activated, ultimately contributing to anxiety.

The microbiome has the ability to deactivate inflammatory genes while activating those that reduce inflammation.

For instance, in terms of gene expression, humans possess approximately 20,000 genes, which constitute about 0.1% of our genetic makeup, whereas the microbiome can express between 2 million and 20 million cells. Consequently, there exists a greater number of foreign cells within the human body compared to human cells. Each gene cell in our body contains identical DNA; however, it is the expression of these genes that determines characteristics such as hair, skin, and teeth. Epigenetics plays a crucial role in regulating gene expression.

Once the microbiome has processed the ingested food, it subsequently releases metabolites, which are small molecules that enter the bloodstream. These metabolites begin to exert epigenetic control over our gene expression, influencing our immune system by signalling whether the consumed substances are beneficial or harmful.

If the food is deemed beneficial, the genes function in a manner consistent with their original design. Conversely, if the ingested item is identified as harmful, gene expression shifts from a healthy state to an unhealthy one, potentially leading to various diseases such as autoimmune disorders, cancer, diabetes, and depression.

I have never received an answer from mainstream medicine as to why the immune system would attack itself. I find it bizarre to reach that conclusion without asking 'why'. Is that not the fundamental principle of all science?

Dr Sebi, Professor Sira, and Professor Ehret have all reported that all disease stems from inflammation in the body, which can lead to oxidative stress. An unhealthy microbiome gives way to free radicals. Free radicals are highly reactive molecules that need to be stabilised; otherwise, they damage the cell membrane, causing the mitochondria in the cell to weaken.

The mitochondria are responsible for 90% of the body's energy. If they are damaged, the body becomes depleted. When the microbiome is affected, every organ in the body, including the brain, can suffer. Free radicals may damage brain cells, resulting in memory and cognitive problems. The liver becomes congested, leading to poor metabolism.

The thyroid is also impacted when the microbiome is dysfunctional. This can lead to the intestinal wall becoming permeable, allowing partially digested and undigested food and bacteria to enter the gut and bloodstream.

The immune system attempts to fend off these intruders, but in doing so, it creates inflammation. This inflammatory response can cause the immune system to mistakenly identify non-intruders as threats if they resemble the actual invaders, potentially leading to autoimmune disease. This cycle results in reduced nutrient absorption.

This theory makes sense: if the immune system is said to be attacking itself but the reason is unknown, why is there no effort to find out? And why is the standard treatment to medicate (essentially switching off the alarm) while the attack is still ongoing?

For example, consider the thyroid, the brain-body juncture. If the thyroid does not produce enough thyroid hormone, it can lead to parasitosis muscle dysfunction. This muscle moves food through the digestive tract via wave-like movements.

The gut is extremely sensitive and relies on enzymes for maintenance. When the gut is exposed to certain products—such as gluten, dairy, soy, meat, pesticides, and processed food—it triggers an inflammatory reaction. Our bodies react negatively to physical, mental, and emotional abuse but respond positively to physical, mental, and emotional support.

We always have the opportunity to support our bodies. Fasting, for example, has been shown to induce autophagy. Autophagy is a process that occurs when cells experience stress or nutrient deprivation. It prompts cells to break down old components and recycle them, cleansing the system naturally by removing non-functioning cells and pathogens.

Additionally, consuming whole foods provided by nature—rather than those manufactured by humans—activates autophagy. This process breaks down damaged cells and bacteria, renewing them to a healthy state. The stomach lining can begin to repair itself in as little as a week for some individuals.

How amazing is that?

Dr Raphael Kellman postulates in his research that even the unhealthiest eaters can experience rapid improvement through these natural processes.

However, if left untreated, this can lead to metabolic endotoxemia, which manifests as leaky gut. (It is important to note that it can take several years for the body to heal due to the long-term damage it has suffered.)

Alternatively, when we consume nutrients that support the microbiome through organic whole foods, as nature intended, and choose to nourish ourselves with positive psychological influences rather than exposing ourselves to negative news and violence, we can foster a healthier existence. The incessant chatter of our egos has contributed significantly to the clutter in both our world and our bodies.

We often complicate matters and fabricate narratives throughout our lives, leading to domination, control, and bullying. This greed, which permeates our society, has been fuelled by these narratives. One manifestation of this greed is the introduction of chemicals into our food supply, resulting in our unintentional dependence on these substances.

We often accept these additives based on the assertions of those behind product labels. When we examine an invention, we typically focus on its functionality, yet our perspective is often limited.

We tend to direct attention to aspects that align with our beliefs while neglecting what may be concealed in the shadows of those beliefs. I observe inventions that do not align with natural principles, such as calories, weight, BMI, and notions of average or ideal sizes.

However, ego-driven thinking is inherently inconsistent and rarely reflects reality. It often promotes a one-size-fits-all approach. If a cell does not receive the necessary nutrients, the body compensates by storing them, which can lead to weight gain.

If your weight looks good, then you appear healthy. However, being informed that you have a healthy weight does not reflect what is inside your body—you could just as easily be weighing rocks.

Your body possesses a profound affinity for your well-being, and when you introduce chemicals into it, these substances are not recognised as food. In an effort to protect you, your body attempts to expel these unidentified substances from your organs. Over time, this process leads to an accumulation of mucus and fat, resulting in an increase in body size.

Consequently, you may be accused of failing to recognise sensations of fullness. This assertion is misleading. Rather, it is your body communicating that it has not received adequate nourishment. What it truly requires is wholesome, natural food, not the chemicals that should be avoided.

The traditional saying, "You are what you eat," has evolved into a more present perspective of simply, "Just eat." Society has often associated slim individuals with healthiness while labelling larger individuals as unhealthy, but this has also led to normalisation.

A common assertion is, "I am a real woman," yet one's identity as a woman is not determined by weight. This narrative contributes to division among individuals and distracts from the real issue at hand: the impact of chemicals on our bodies. Our bodies do not recognise made-up labels. They communicate with us through reactions, feelings, and emotions. Chemicals serve their intended purpose, causing effects that often neglect the body's well-being, resulting in side effects.

When individuals experience a quick resolution to what they perceive as a problem, they may feel satisfied. However, this focus on immediate results obscures the underlying issues. For instance, taking a painkiller for a headache addresses the symptom, but the potential harm to the stomach remains unacknowledged.

Although the immediate relief may seem beneficial, the eventual consequences of such actions can lead to further complications, necessitating additional medication. Professor Tim Spector adds that depression and anxiety are intrinsically linked to the food we eat.

This is a shadow that is also overlooked in food that is wrapped up in a programme of "juicy, flavoursome, mouth-watering yumminess." These are the chemicals and antibiotics (mould) you consume when eating a product dressed up in colourful, shiny packaging, happy faces, and crispy, cracking, and crunchy noises that tell you in advance how "yummy" the chemicals, fat, sugar, salt, and mucus-forming products are going to taste.

We are drawn in by all kinds of stories because we are directed by a spotlight, but we rarely look at what is behind the spotlight. What is in the shadow, or the implications of what is in the shadow, is often not fully considered or is ignored.

We often do not validate or love our bodies; instead, we allow egoic thinking to use them.

Man-made Provider

Cally Means (2024) articulates the notion that both the food and medical industries foster dependency and poor health, as it aligns with their commercial interests and overarching narratives. Means reports perspectives that oppose those in mainstream media regarding treatment and the medical model. He asserts that the medical sector has remained complicit, drawing lessons from those who benefit financially from this situation.

Means refers to this phenomenon as the "Devil's Bargain." This troubling trend can be traced back to 1909 when heroin was the fourth most prescribed medication, astonishingly administered to nearly every infant in the nation and marketed by Bayer as a remedy for difficult behaviour.

The significant progress in medical treatments over the last century can be attributed primarily to the swift advancements in chemistry and pharmacology. Throughout this time, countless compounds synthesised in laboratories were evaluated for their therapeutic potential, with those deemed effective subsequently manufactured for commercial use.

Public acceptance and the prevalence of any particular drug have typically been influenced by the medical community. Many newly introduced compounds were utilised only briefly, often supplanted by alternatives that demonstrated greater efficacy or fewer adverse effects.

The case of heroin (diacetylmorphine) stands out as particularly exceptional. Initially celebrated as a miraculous medication, it garnered enthusiastic support from healthcare professionals. However, the harmful consequences of the drug soon came to light. Despite many physicians ceasing to prescribe heroin and cautioning against its reckless use, demand for the substance persisted, making it challenging to limit its consumption.

Means explains that John Davison Rockefeller Sr. was an American business magnate and philanthropist. At the age of 16, he took on the role of an assistant bookkeeper and entered into various business partnerships starting at the age of 20, with a focus on the oil refining industry.

In 1870, Rockefeller established the Standard Oil Company, which he managed until 1897, maintaining his position as its largest shareholder. Following his retirement, he dedicated his resources and efforts to philanthropic endeavours, particularly in the fields of education, healthcare, higher education, and the modernisation of the Southern United States.

He was instrumental in the inception of the modern pharmaceutical industry, primarily by exploring the potential applications of oil-based by-products. Rockefeller emerged as a significant benefactor to educational institutions, including Johns

Hopkins and other early medical schools, with the aim of establishing evidence-based medicine.

This approach categorised diseases into distinct silos, which impeded communication and collaboration among medical professionals. The objective was to enable physicians to either perform surgeries or prescribe medications. Such a medical paradigm was considered radical at the time, as predominant medical theories and treatments were more holistic in nature.

Rockefeller, however, advocated for identifying symptoms and prescribing drugs accordingly. The contemporary medical education system, characterised by residency programmes and specialised fields, originated from this concept. The primary motivation behind this structure was not to enhance the health of the American populace but rather to promote the sale of pharmaceutical drugs.

This framework was articulated by Flexner, an associate of Rockefeller, and presented to Congress in the Flexner Report of 1909, which laid the groundwork for evidence-based medicine. Consequently, this became the sole type of medicine that the U.S. government would support and disseminate.

One of the major advancements during this period was the promotion of antibiotics alongside other medications. Antibiotics were associated with victory in World War II, presenting themselves as a rapid solution to health issues. One of the earliest chronic conditions identified was pregnancy during the war, and in the 1950s, the introduction of the birth control pill was quickly recognised by medical leaders as a lucrative business model, as it is a medication that female patients are likely to continue using long-term.

Arthur Sackler completed his residency in psychiatry at the Creedmoor Psychiatric Centre. From 1949 to 1954, he served as the director of research at the Creedmoor Institute for Psychobiological Studies, where he focused on biological psychiatry. Throughout his career, Sackler co-authored numerous papers in the fields of neuroendocrinology, psychiatry, and experimental medicine. He is recognised as the first physician to use ultrasound as a diagnostic instrument.

The Sackler brothers pursued their studies in Scotland, became psychiatrists, and joined the research team at Creedmoor. They collaborated closely with Johan H. W. Van Ophuijsen, the director, who was regarded by Arthur Sackler as "Freud's favourite disciple."

Mortimer Sackler's grandfather began to explore the potential for the creation of more chronic health issues. He focused on Valium, which gained significant popularity during the 1960s and 1970s; it is documented that over 30% of women were using Valium during this period.

This medication was marketed through advertisements as a "happy pill," despite its addictive properties. The Sackler family operated the largest network of medical journals, disseminating information that influenced the medical community. They effectively secured government support, allowing them to establish new disease categories, including menopause and anxiety, among others. This gradual approach led to the fragmentation of diseases and the development of specific drugs for each condition.

The implication is that working within a large corporation can lead to a sense of isolation, making it easy to become disconnected from reality.

Means postulates that the Sackler family's influence on the medical system was profound, as they sought to extend the trust established in acute care post-World War II to chronic conditions. In the 1960s, nearly 0% of the U.S. healthcare budget was allocated to chronic illnesses; today, that figure exceeds 90%, indicating a significant shift towards chronic care.

The expansion of the chronic disease sector has considerably grown the healthcare industry, yet it has largely been deemed a failure. Means highlights that the corrupt legal framework established in the 1900s remains unchanged. The Flexner Report continues to serve as a foundational document in medicine today, compelling students to select from one of 42 specialties—a system devised by John Rockefeller that divides the human body into 42 distinct parts.

Instead of addressing the root causes of overall health problems, the medical model focuses on treating one of the 42 parts separately, allowing for more treatments or drugs to be administered—thus creating a profitable medical model and a "profitable patient," which is good for business. It is misleading to tell a patient they have multiple separate issues when, in reality, these conditions may be interconnected. However, this is not what is taught.

John Rockefeller's faith was profoundly influenced by his Baptist upbringing. He perceived his achievements as a blessing from God and felt a moral obligation to utilise his fortune for the benefit of others. His philanthropic efforts included substantial contributions to numerous charities and institutions, such as the University of Chicago and the Rockefeller Foundation, both of which continue to operate today. Paradoxically, he agreed with the Darwinian theory and postulated that the growth of a large business is merely the survival of the fittest.

Here, we can see the change in the Hippocratic Oath, which originally stated, "I will give no deadly medicine to even those that ask," compared to the modern-day oath, which is now deemed a guideline. The original oath focused on caring for one another, whereas today, the focus is on money.

The Industrial Revolution marks a significant period in modern history, characterised by the transition from an agricultural and artisanal economy to one primarily governed by industrial production and machine manufacturing. This wave of technological advancements brought about innovative methods of labour and lifestyle, leading to profound societal transformations.

However, my research has revealed that this revolution was not solely beneficial to humanity. We are not only the workers but also the providers, paying with both our minds and bodies to sustain those who worship money. Here, I have found that money itself is not evil—because none of us truly possess it. Instead, we hold only "I owe you" notes, mere "promissory notes."

On 30 October 2017, *The New Yorker* published an extensive exposé concerning Mortimer Sackler, Purdue Pharma, and the Sackler family as a whole. The article linked the business strategies of Raymond and Arthur Sackler with the emergence of direct pharmaceutical marketing, ultimately connecting them to the opioid addiction crisis in the United States. It suggested that Sackler bears a degree of moral responsibility for the opioid epidemic.

In 2019, *The New York Times* published an article confirming that Sackler instructed company officials in 2008 to evaluate the company's performance not only by the volume of drug doses sold but also by the potency of those doses. This information was corroborated by legally obtained documents related to a new lawsuit filed in June by Massachusetts Attorney General Maura Healey.

The *Times* reported that the lawsuit alleged Purdue Pharma and members of the Sackler family were aware that placing patients on high dosages of OxyContin for extended periods heightened the risks of severe side effects, including addiction. Nevertheless, they advocated for higher dosages because more potent pain medications yielded greater profits for both the company and the Sacklers.

More recently, on 21 October 2024, I watched a U.S. congressional hearing titled:

"Dishonest Director TORCHED for Repeatedly LYING at Congressional Hearing."

The hearing began with James Daniel Jordan, an American politician currently serving his ninth term in the U.S. House of Representatives. Dr Wenstrup, the chairman, introduced Mr Jordan, who immediately questioned Dr Walensky, the CDC Director.

"Why did you and the Biden Administration mislead the American people?"

Dr Walensky asked Mr Jordan to elaborate. He did so by referring to a statement Dr Walensky had made on 29 March 2021:

"Vaccinated people do not carry the virus; vaccinated people don't get sick. We got that information from a clinical trial but also from real-world data."

He proceeded to highlight a number of statements made by Dr Walensky that were inaccurate. Dr Walensky responded with a sweeping answer, stating that the information she provided on 29 March 2021 was "generally accurate." Mr Jordan pressed further, asking, "Why not be truthful?"

"We pay your salary. The government is supposed to be of the people, for the people, by the people."

Mr Jordan then referred to another statement Dr Walensky had made six weeks later:

"If you were to get infected post-vaccination, you can't give it to anyone else."

He asked, "Was that accurate?" to which she again replied, "Generally true."

Mr Jordan countered, "But we know that was not accurate."

He then asked, "Was it our tax dollars that you used in the lab in China?"

Dr Walensky responded, "That is something you would have to speak to NIH about" (National Institutes of Health).

Mr Jordan replied, "Our tax dollars were used. It sure looked like it was 'gain of function' research. It sure looked like it actually came from the lab, and we've had several federal agencies say that's, in fact, where the virus originated."

He then referred back to statements made by the Biden Administration, adding that the public was also told that the virus offered no natural immunity. Summarising, Mr Jordan pointed out that seven different statements had since been proven untrue. The hearing continued with further questioning of Dr Walensky and the Biden Administration.

Dr Wenstrup then introduced Ms Greene from Georgia.

Ms Greene reiterated that Dr Walensky had previously stated that COVID-19 vaccines were "safe and effective." She pointed to 1.5 million VAERS (Vaccine Adverse Event Reporting System) reports, which also included 35,000 deaths allegedly associated with the COVID-19 vaccine.

Ms Greene stated that many Americans felt the CDC and Dr Walensky had ignored these reports. She noted that in late 2020, Pfizer's COVID-19 vaccine was approved, followed by a federal mandate in 2021.

"For example, federal contractors and employees—90% of the 3.5 million people employed—received at least one dose of the vaccine. Vaccine cards were also implemented in Democrat-run cities across the country, essentially making vaccination a requirement to participate in society."

She further reported that in 2021, COVID-19-related reports surged to number one in the VAERS database, reaching 728,829 reports, while the second-highest—Zostavax (the shingles vaccine)—had just over 14,000. Ms Greene stated that VAERS reports continued to increase.

Ms Greene also addressed how much the American taxpayer was forced to pay Pfizer and Moderna for vaccines. The government paid Pfizer and Moderna in 2020, 2021, and 2022. Pfizer received $15.27 billion, while Moderna received $9.99 billion. And they certainly got a return on the American taxpayers' investment—because in 2022, Pfizer saw a 23% increase in revenue, but in 2021, they doubled their income with a 95% increase in revenue.

Moderna's revenue skyrocketed as well. In 2020, they saw a staggering 1,238% increase, and in 2021, their revenue surged by 2,200%, thanks to the American taxpayer. Government funding flowed into these big pharmaceutical companies for the production of vaccines. It is quite remarkable that Pfizer, on a global scale, went from $190 billion at the beginning of 2021 to an astonishing $330 billion worldwide by the end of the year.

Ms Greene sarcastically thanked the CDC and Dr Walensky, who had assured the public that vaccines were "safe and effective." She also addressed the advice given to pregnant women to receive the COVID-19 vaccine, revealing a massive increase in miscarriages and stillbirths. Unfortunately, Dr Walensky's response was to rebut these findings without offering any real substance.

It has come to my attention that, despite experiencing disappointments in our healthcare system and suffering due to the harmful actions of those we rely on for assistance, we continue to exhibit a form of Stockholm syndrome—placing our trust in individuals who have deceived us and failed to meet our expectations.

The verbal abuse, assaults, and intimidation directed at individuals who chose not to receive the COVID-19 vaccine— coming from medical professionals, government officials, and the media—have been pervasive. Yet, I have yet to encounter a single apology for these actions. There also appears to be an increasing trend towards vaccinating the human body to the point of rendering it incapable.

Food Companies

Smoking has been a practice observed in various forms since ancient civilisations. Evidence suggests that tobacco and different hallucinogenic substances were utilised in shamanistic rituals across America as early as 5000 BC, with origins traced back to the Andes regions of Peru and Ecuador.

Initially, smoking likely stemmed from the incense-burning ceremonies conducted by shamans, but it later evolved into a practice for enjoyment and social interaction. The act of smoking tobacco and hallucinogenic drugs was often employed to induce trances and facilitate communication with the spiritual realm.

Calley Means (2024) has reported that in the early 1900s, the tobacco industry developed an ideal product. Cigarettes became easy to manufacture, affordable, and highly addictive. By 1910, the United States was producing millions of cigarettes annually—a figure that surged to 123 billion by 1930—demonstrating the industry's profitability.

However, this success was overshadowed when medical professionals identified a direct correlation between smoking and cancer.

Edward Bernays, renowned for his expertise in propaganda, utilised his skills to garner American support for the war. He began his work with the Committee on Public Information, where he influenced public sentiment through rallies. Pro-war materials, such as brochures titled *Uncle Sam Needs You*, were widely distributed. Bernays captured the attention of President Woodrow Wilson, who was impressed by his efforts and invited him to the Paris Peace Conference.

Means describes how Bernays recognised the potential of role models as influencers, leading individuals to aspire to what these figures represented. In the realm of health and nutrition, society often looks to doctors, conditioned to believe that they have superior knowledge. Bernays effectively used role models from various sectors to promote the products he was advocating to the public, earning him a reputation as a propaganda pioneer.

He leveraged the products he endorsed as a narrative device about human behaviour. For instance, smoking was portrayed as a symbol of masculinity. To market tobacco to women and increase sales, he crafted a new narrative.

During a time when women were advocating for equal rights, advertising suggested that smoking was a means to reclaim power and freedom, positioning women as equal to men. This strategy proved remarkably effective, as women began expressing their equality through smoking. As a result, the tobacco industry experienced a significant expansion, with sales tripling within a year—transforming a harmful, addictive substance into a symbol of liberation.

Nevertheless, challenges persisted for tobacco companies, which sought to project an image of concern for their customers. They funded research that claimed there was no definitive evidence linking cigarettes to health issues, framing cancer cases as anomalies. In response to growing scrutiny, tobacco companies developed "healthier" cigarette options.

However, as television advertising for cigarettes was eventually banned, these companies turned to celebrity endorsements and sponsorship of sporting events. The film industry became a platform for cigarette advertising, facilitating expansion into developing nations and targeting younger audiences—resulting in the industry reaching $818 billion in 2019.

Subsequently, Bernays applied the same propaganda techniques he had used for wartime efforts to the food industry, framing his initiatives as public relations campaigns. His remarkable ability to influence public opinion enabled him to persuade doctors to endorse the idea that a more substantial breakfast was beneficial. This led to the promotion of pork products, including bacon and eggs, as breakfast staples.

In the 1990s, two prominent food corporations, R.J. Reynolds and Philip Morris, took significant steps in response to the Surgeon General's declaration in the 1980s regarding the potential dangers of cigarettes. Faced with increasing regulatory scrutiny on tobacco products, these financially robust companies began acquiring food enterprises as a strategic manoeuvre.

Philip Morris made a notable acquisition in 1988 when it purchased Kraft Foods for $12.9 billion, followed by the acquisition of Nabisco Holdings Corporation for $14.9 billion—thereby establishing one of the largest food conglomerates globally. Meanwhile, R.J. Reynolds merged with Nabisco Holdings Corporation in 1985.

The overarching objective of these companies was to leverage their expertise in creating addictive products from cigarettes and apply similar strategies to the food industry. Means stipulates that they employed scientists who had previously developed the same active chemicals used in cigarettes to enhance food products, thereby reaching consumers worldwide and cultivating a market of unsuspecting individuals who would become dependent on their products.

This approach proved to be highly profitable, fostering lifelong consumer loyalty. The food products available to consumers were essentially the result of scientific experimentation, leading to the prevalence of processed and ultra-processed foods.

Means describes how, subsequently, these corporations altered their strategies within the food sector, influencing consumer behaviour and manipulating institutional trust. They established a food pyramid and allegedly engaged in unethical practices, including providing financial incentives to the FDA and the United States Department of Agriculture (USDA), as well as to Harvard University and Stanford University, to downplay the effects of these products. They even produced a report asserting that sugar does not contribute to obesity.

In 1992, they lobbied for the food pyramid, which claimed that animal-based fats were detrimental to health while promoting carbohydrates as beneficial.

Due to our inherent trust in labels—particularly those from medical institutions regarding health and nutrition—we have adapted our diets to include processed and ultra-processed foods, effectively consuming chemicals instead.

The food pyramid served as a marketing tool for processed foods, suggesting that carbohydrates and sugar were acceptable dietary choices.

The components found in processed foods include refined sugars and processed grains, which often lack fiber and function similarly to sugar.

Additionally, seed oils—a by-product of oil production pioneered by John Rockefeller—are utilised as lubricants and are incorporated into both processed and ultra-processed foods. For instance, when consuming a packet of crisps, it is possible that they have been fried in oils originally intended for engine lubrication, yet repurposed for human consumption.

Currently, adults and parents not only consume these chemicals but also feed them to their children, who now ingest approximately 70% of their diet from processed foods. These products, developed by the tobacco industry to create addiction in children, would provoke outrage if we witnessed a child smoking a cigarette.

Yet, we often exhibit either blind acceptance or wilful ignorance when we allow our children to consume addictive chemicals that contribute to their physical and mental ailments. This consumption of a toxic cocktail of chemicals disrupts our cellular health, leading to the increasing prevalence of illness in society.

We are ingesting substances that our bodies are not biologically equipped to process—substances that did not exist a century ago—all for the profit of certain businesses.

Water

The Earth is predominantly composed of water, which is essential for all forms of life, including humans. Our existence, as well as that of the planet, is fundamentally dependent on water. However, rather than consuming pure water, we often opt for flavoured beverages.

This choice leads to a persistent state of dehydration, depriving our bodies of the life-sustaining properties of pure water. This can result in various health issues and diminished brain and organ function. Water, a compound formed from hydrogen and oxygen, is both abundant and essential. It is tasteless and odourless at room temperature and possesses a remarkable ability to dissolve numerous substances.

This solvent capability is crucial for living organisms, as it is believed that life originated in the aquatic environments of Earth's oceans. Organisms depend on water-based solutions, such as blood and digestive fluids, for vital biological processes. Water is also present on other celestial bodies within and beyond our solar system.

As the most effective solvent on Earth, water can exist in three states: gas, liquid, and solid. Remarkably, it can even defy gravity, as evidenced by plants that penetrate through tarmac due to their water content.

Water is composed of atoms, which are the smallest units of elements like oxygen and hydrogen. These atoms combine to form molecules, with a water molecule consisting of two hydrogen (H) atoms and one oxygen (O) atom, hence the designation H_2O. A single drop of water contains billions of these molecules.

Furthermore, water behaves similarly to the nervous system in response to stimuli. Each water molecule is a dipole, with one end carrying a positive charge and the other a negative charge. This polarity allows molecules to attract one another, forming clusters. Within these clusters, water retains information from any substances it encounters, as these substances leave a trace within the water.

Research indicates that if a region is susceptible to trauma, the effects of that trauma are retained in the water, as water is believed to possess memory. Any external influences that water encounters imprint this memory onto it. Professor Rustum Roy from Pennsylvania State University likens water to computer memory.

In January 2005, a group of Russian biophysicists travelled to Venezuela to collect water samples after learning that Roraima is referred to as the "mother of all water." The scientists hypothesised that this water had never been in direct contact with humans, making Venezuela the sole location on Earth where such pristine, untouched water existed—until the biophysicists interacted with it.

The Pemon Indian tribe, who live in deprivation, exhibit happiness and longevity, expressing a strong desire to remain untouched by Western civilisation. Professor Kotkov's assistant created a device capable of assessing the energetics of water, based on the curling effect. When an object enters a strong electromagnetic field, it begins to emit light; the more energy the object possesses, the brighter it shines.

The Venezuelan water was compared to standard drinking water, revealing that the pure, virgin water was 40,000 times more active than its ordinary counterpart. This water had an immediate energising effect on the body, which was evident in the scientific team, despite their brief stay of less than a week. Dr Korotkov utilised a specialised instrument to measure the energy levels of each team member at the base of Roraima and again two days after they reached the summit.

Professor Kotkov described his findings as remarkable, noting that the energy field of individuals at sea level displayed numerous breaks and irregularities, which contrasted sharply with the significant changes observed in those who had ascended to the Roraima summit.

Water is considered a living entity, and according to Viktor Schauberger, this entity can perish if subjected to improper treatment. Schauberger posited that water originates in the forest, descends as rain, and filters through rocks, accumulating minerals and trace elements until it reaches a spring, prepared to sustain life.

This process is influenced by the natural flow of water versus artificial manipulation. Our lack of awareness leads us to neglect the treatment of water. We direct water through straight channels and artificial systems, whereas nature does not conform to straight lines; such lines are a human construct. We disregard the natural course of water. Spiral patterns and arrangements are prevalent in our environment, representing formations that embody constant change.

To establish a system that serves water effectively, we must replicate the formations found in nature, allowing water to breathe and pulsate rhythmically. This process energises, restructures, and oxygenates the water while eliminating any detrimental information it may have absorbed.

The water that we convey through pipelines travels in straight lines and at right angles, disrupting its natural structure. As a result, the water appears in various forms, such as crystals that are misshapen, losing their inherent beauty and symmetry.

Dr Masaru Emoto, a Japanese water researcher, has been studying crystal formation for over 15 years. His findings indicate that water crystals typically exhibit a hexagonal shape, while water that is lifeless or less vibrant manifests in distorted forms. This phenomenon is particularly evident in urban water sources, where the water absorbs negative information from pollution and human activity.

Furthermore, the addition of chemicals to water correlates with a decrease in crystal formation. Dr Emoto's conclusions align with those of Professors Kotkov and Schauberger. Max Planck stated that everything is a wave. When we inscribe a word on a piece of paper and place it near water, we can observe a transformation in the water's structure.

This change signifies a metamorphosis of the water itself, influenced by the frequencies emitted by the written word. When water becomes unhealthy or dies, it reacts adversely to devices such as mobile phones, televisions, microwave ovens, and computers. This occurs because everything in the universe operates on vibrations, which require resonance.

In the quantum realm, minuscule particles resonate with one another, affirming their existence. We can reaffirm the reality of objects through this concept of resonance. Since all living organisms are fundamentally composed of water, we can observe how a negative environment and harmful words can lead to feelings of illness and energy depletion, while a positive environment and uplifting words can enhance our vitality.

Additionally, sunlight invigorates water, which explains why we feel revitalised in the sun. Water that flows through a natural spring under sunlight hydrates and nourishes our bodies, in contrast to water confined in dark pipes.

Research indicates that human beings consist of approximately 70% to 90% water. To maintain essential bodily functions, an adult should consume between two and two and a half litres of water daily. Additionally, around one and a half litres of water is absorbed through the skin during activities such as showering or bathing.

It is remarkable how water never leaks out of the body when you cut yourself. The only time water is expelled is during cleaning or to cool us down through perspiration.

Water serves as a fundamental connection between all entities on Earth, acting as the medium through which nature operates. It facilitates the exchange of vast amounts of information that binds us all together.

Maintaining proper hydration is vital for our overall health; however, many individuals find it challenging to achieve sufficient hydration levels. Although it is widely recognised that a daily intake of at least two litres of water is necessary, a considerable number of people do not reach this goal.

The interdependence of bodily functions is significant, with hydration being a critical factor. For example, the processes of skin renewal and rejuvenation cannot proceed effectively in a dehydrated state. Regrettably, many individuals frequently experience dehydration.

Increasing water consumption is crucial; however, it frequently entails the introduction of various substances found in tap water, including fluoride, chlorine, oestrogen, and other chemicals. It is vital to recognise the adverse effects associated with these components of tap water and to seek out healthier, cost-effective alternatives.

For instance, fluoride is incorporated into tap water as a preventive measure against tooth decay, even though it does not enhance the quality or safety of the water. This treatment is provided without informed consent, lacks proper dosage regulation, and is not evaluated for its appropriateness for each individual.

In adults, roughly 50–60% of fluoride consumed is eliminated by the kidneys daily, while the remainder is deposited in calcifying tissues such as bones and the pineal gland. Children, on the other hand, tend to retain even greater proportions of fluoride in their skeletal system.

Recent research indicates that the advantages of fluoride for dental health are largely topical rather than systemic. This implies that any beneficial effects of fluoride on dental care arise from its direct application to the teeth rather than from ingestion.

In light of these findings, there is no rationale for the consumption of fluoride. The fluoride contained in toothpaste or mouthwash, which is applied directly to the teeth and subsequently rinsed away, is seen as adequate for maintaining dental health. However, most fluoride-based products can also kill the microbiome in our mouths due to their chemical ingredients.

The Environmental Protection Agency (EPA) has recognised fluoride as one of approximately 100 substances with "substantial evidence of developmental neurotoxicity." A report published in March 2014 by *The Lancet*, a prestigious medical journal, classified fluoride as a neurotoxin, categorising it alongside arsenic, lead, and mercury.

A multitude of studies conducted in countries such as China, Iran, India, and Mexico have established a link between fluoride exposure and reduced IQ, with a total of 33 studies reported to date. Furthermore, fluoride accumulates in significant quantities within the pineal gland and has been shown to influence thyroid function, to the extent that it has been employed as a treatment for hyperthyroidism.

Additionally, fluoride has been linked to arthritic symptoms, with early signs of skeletal fluorosis resembling those of arthritis. Tests have revealed a significant correlation between the fluoridation of water supplies and cortical bone defects, as well as the frequency of bone fractures.

There is also evidence suggesting that fluoride may contribute to Alzheimer's disease and other forms of dementia. The presence of aluminium in the brain has a strong association with these conditions, and fluoride impairs the barrier that prevents metals from entering the brain.

The ongoing discussion surrounding the potential risks associated with fluoride suggests that the concerns raised should be sufficient to encourage individuals to reconsider the consumption of fluoridated water. Water authorities are often reticent in disclosing which sources contain added fluoride, complicating efforts to determine the actual number of individuals impacted by fluoridation. Consequently, it is prudent to approach the information provided by these authorities with a degree of scepticism.

While the list of potential harms caused by fluoride continues, the aforementioned points should be enough to question why we place our trust in those we do not know when it comes to our health. Water boards are not forthcoming about which supplies have fluoride added, making it difficult to ascertain the true number of people affected by fluoridation. Therefore, it is advisable to exercise caution when relying on their information regarding fluoridation.

Chlorine

Chlorine is a hazardous and corrosive gas that can be transformed into a liquid state through the process of compression. This liquid form is subsequently introduced into drinking water and swimming pools to eradicate bacteria and various microorganisms.

You may have noticed an unpleasant taste or odour in tap water, which can be attributed to the chlorine routinely added to it.

Beyond its application in water treatment, chlorine is also employed in the production of antifreeze, pesticides, and bleach. While the Drinking Water Inspectorate assures that the residual chlorine levels in tap water are within safe limits, concerns may arise not from chlorine itself but from its reaction with natural organic matter. This reaction leads to the formation of Disinfection By-Products (DBPs) such as trihalomethanes and haloacetic acids.

A study conducted in Iowa in 1997 revealed that postmenopausal women living in regions with elevated DBP levels exhibited nearly double the incidence of colon cancer compared to those in areas with lower DBP concentrations.

Since the early 1990s, there has been a growing body of evidence suggesting a possible association between chlorinated water and bladder cancer. Research indicates that the consumption of tap water during pregnancy may elevate the risk of significant heart or brain abnormalities in the developing foetus. A comprehensive study involving nearly 400,000 infants demonstrated a distinct correlation between chlorination by-products and the incidence of specific birth defects.

Numerous epidemiological investigations, including those conducted by the National Cancer Institute and other research bodies, have established a link between the chlorination of drinking water and an increased likelihood of bladder cancer. Additional studies have indicated a potential rise in the occurrence of Hodgkin's disease, colorectal cancer, oesophageal cancer, and breast cancer.

The data indicates that women diagnosed with breast cancer exhibit organochlorine levels (by-products of chlorination) in their breast tissue that are 50–60% higher than those found in women without breast cancer.

Moreover, certain animal studies have associated chlorination with reduced sperm counts, male infertility, and various circulatory problems.

Water authorities regularly invite stakeholders to examine the latest favourable reports concerning the quality of their water supplies. Nevertheless, they refrain from revealing the concentrations of oestrogen and other hormones due to insufficient testing. Ethinyl oestradiol, a synthetic form of oestrogen present in contraceptive medications and hormone replacement therapies, is contaminating water supplies, as it is not entirely removed during sewage treatment processes.

A range of symptoms and health issues associated with oestrogen dominance includes various cancers, premenopausal bone density loss, accelerated ageing, osteoporosis, weight gain, insomnia, cognitive decline, allergies, fatigue, fibrocystic breast conditions, breast sensitivity, hair loss, irregular menstrual cycles, gallbladder diseases, mood fluctuations, depression, autoimmune disorders, headaches, increased blood clotting, thyroid dysfunction, hypoglycaemia, polycystic ovary syndrome, premenstrual syndrome (PMS), reduced libido, infertility, sluggish metabolism, dry eyes, irritability, early onset of menstruation, uterine fibroids, uterine cancer, endometrial cancer, water retention, copper excess, magnesium deficiency, and zinc deficiency, among others.

Furthermore, hormones from livestock and synthetic chemicals from various origins also contaminate water supplies, with current removal methods proving inadequate. The effects of these substances on human health are still largely uncharted.

Toxic Environment

From the preceding discussion, it is clear that you are now familiar with the concept of a toxic environment. The discomfort experienced in the body arises from the poisoning of cells, leading to toxicity or heightened sensitivity.

In one of her medical lectures, Patricia Caine illustrated the phenomenon of toxic cells by presenting slides that depicted cells in a toxic state. Various toxins—including lead, mercury, mould, herbicides, pesticides, and chemicals found in food and pharmaceuticals—contribute to this condition.

The slides demonstrated that the cell membranes become compromised due to saturation with these toxins. This prevents the cells from effectively eliminating them, leading to persistent accumulation. When cells encounter irritants such as scents, food, temperature fluctuations, or chemicals, this triggers the release of toxins into the bloodstream, exacerbating disease within the body.

Molecules that are lipophilic (attracted to fats) and hydrophilic (attracted to water) can attach to various components within the body. This allows them to bypass any cell they encounter, as they interact with the fatty materials that constitute every membrane in the body or blend into aqueous solutions.

Additionally, sensitivity occurs when the nervous system is exposed to a multitude of stimuli, including sounds, lighting, electromagnetic fields (EMFs) from devices like mobile phones, laptops, tablets, video games, and smart meters, as well as touch, food, odours, and chemicals found in household and personal care products (such as shampoos, creams, and toothpaste). This sensitivity can manifest as allergies, heightened startle responses, irritability, or fear.

Furthermore, exposure to *Bartonella* and mould can sensitise cells, leading to the release of significant amounts of histamine. This may result in symptoms such as flushing, palpitations, abdominal pain, diarrhoea, and/or sweating. Other potential reactions include cognitive impairment, muscle twitching or jerking motions, pseudo-seizures, and fatigue.

The nervous system reacts to prolonged exposure to a hostile environment, resulting in a state of dis-ease and discomfort. Sensitivity can be heightened when toxins are removed, as these toxins contribute to overall toxicity, and sensitivity reflects the experience of that toxicity. The objective is to reduce sensitivity first, allowing for the effective management of the toxins. Treatment options include binders for mould toxins, such as bentonite clay, activated charcoal, and cholestyramine.

It is estimated that 75% of the population possesses a genetic structure that enables the elimination of certain toxins, such as mould, through antibodies. Conversely, individuals lacking these antibodies have toxins directed to the liver, lungs, gastrointestinal tract, skin, or lymphatic system for detoxification. If these systems become overwhelmed with toxins and are unable to perform their detoxification functions, the entire system may become compromised.

Wilful Ignorance.

Those who do not consider diverse viewpoints and instead cling to a limited perspective often sustain outdated narratives of misunderstanding, such as asserting, "It's all in your mind," or trivialising concerns as psychosomatic. This attitude is not rooted in scientific investigation. The essence of science lies in the pursuit of uncovering the unknown and discovering precise answers, rather than remaining in ignorance and constructing subjective narratives.

The analysis of environmental toxins that were nearly absent over fifty years ago reveals a troubling reality: the chemicals we now consume and are exposed to are having a profound impact on our health. This is particularly evident in the rising prevalence of conditions once deemed uncommon, such as Lyme disease and mould exposure, which are frequently associated with antibiotic use.

One does not need an advanced degree to recognise the transformations in our surroundings. We can no longer afford to deny, ignore, or overlook the exploitation of the human body as a means of generating profit through the use of chemicals and electronics. It seems we are being treated akin to livestock. Such treatment is unacceptable for animals and should be equally intolerable for humans, as we confront the negative repercussions of prioritising commercial interests over our well-being.

The Industrial Revolution in Britain commenced approximately in 1760 and continued until roughly 1820–1840. This era marked a significant transformation in Great Britain, characterised by numerous technological advancements and architectural innovations. My inquiry is whether this phenomenon was driven by greatness or greed. Are we just a cog in the industry?

How Do Hormones and Antibiotics Impact Animals?

Doris Lin, an animal rights attorney and the Director of Legal and Government Affairs for the Animal Protection League of New Jersey, stated in 2018 that numerous individuals are taken aback to learn that antibiotics and growth hormones are commonly administered to farmed animals. This practice raises significant issues regarding both animal welfare and public health.

In factory farming operations, there is little regard for the well-being of animals, whether considered as a group or as individuals. The animals are viewed primarily as commodities, and substances like rBGH are utilised to enhance the profitability of these enterprises.

Recombinant bovine growth hormone (rBGH), also referred to as recombinant bovine somatotropin (rBST), is an artificial form of a hormone that is naturally synthesised by cows in their pituitary glands. Dairy producers utilise rBST to enhance the milk yield of their cattle.

The speed at which an animal reaches slaughter weight or the volume of milk it produces directly correlates with the profitability of the operation. In the United States, approximately two-thirds of beef cattle are administered growth hormones, while around 22 percent of dairy cows receive hormones to enhance milk yield.

Recombinant bovine growth hormone (rBGH) is known to increase milk production in cows; however, its safety for both humans and animals remains a subject of debate. Moreover, the use of this synthetic hormone has been linked to a higher occurrence of mastitis, an infection of the udder that can lead to the presence of blood and pus in the milk.

In contrast, the European Union has prohibited the use of hormones in beef cattle and has conducted research indicating that hormone residues persist in the meat. Due to health concerns affecting both humans and animals, countries such as Japan, Canada, Australia, and the European Union have all banned the use of recombinant bovine growth hormone (rBGH), although it continues to be administered to cows in the United States.

Furthermore, the European Union has prohibited the importation of meat from animals treated with hormones, resulting in no beef imports from the United States.

To address mastitis and other illnesses, cows and various farmed animals are routinely administered antibiotics as a preventive strategy. When a single animal within a herd or flock is diagnosed with a disease, the entire group is treated with the medication, typically incorporated into their feed or water, as diagnosing and treating individual animals would be prohibitively expensive. Consequently, healthy cows are receiving antibiotics unnecessarily, which introduces additional health risks.

The overuse of antibiotics raises significant concerns due to the emergence of antibiotic-resistant bacterial strains. While antibiotics effectively eliminate most bacteria, they leave behind resistant strains that can proliferate rapidly in the absence of competition.

These resistant bacteria can then disseminate throughout the farm and potentially to humans who interact with the animals or consume animal products. This concern is not unfounded, as antibiotic-resistant strains of salmonella have already been detected in animal products within the human food supply.

Another issue arises from the use of "subtherapeutic" doses of antibiotics, which are administered to promote weight gain in animals. Although the mechanism by which low doses of antibiotics facilitate weight gain remains unclear, this practice has been prohibited in the European Union and Canada, yet it remains legal in the United States.

The World Health Organisation advocates for the necessity of prescriptions for antibiotics administered to farmed animals.

Additionally, numerous countries have prohibited the use of recombinant bovine growth hormone (rBGH) and the application of subtherapeutic doses of antibiotics. However, these measures appear to primarily focus on human health and fail to take into account the rights of animals.

How do hormones and antibiotics impact Humans?

A number of medical professionals express uncertainty regarding the origins of autoimmune diseases and the reasons for their higher prevalence in women compared to men. One hypothesis suggests that elevated hormone levels in women, particularly due to the use of contraceptive pills or hormone replacement therapy during reproductive years, may increase susceptibility to these conditions.

When the body detects a threat from a virus or infection, the immune system activates and mounts an attack, known as an immune response. Occasionally, this response inadvertently targets healthy cells and tissues, leading to the development of autoimmune diseases.

Some theorists propose that genetic factors contribute to the onset of autoimmune diseases, although researchers have yet to fully elucidate the mechanisms involved. For instance, having a family history of conditions such as lupus or multiple sclerosis (MS) can elevate an individual's risk of developing these diseases. It is also observed that certain families may have multiple members affected by various autoimmune disorders. Nevertheless, genetics alone cannot account for the emergence of autoimmune diseases.

Dr Ana-Maria Orbai emphasises the significance of genes while acknowledging their limitations. "While genetics play a crucial role, they are not the sole factor," she states. "It is possible to have relatives with lupus or multiple sclerosis and never experience these conditions yourself. Furthermore, one might test positive for lupus-specific DNA without actually having the disease."

The onset of autoimmune diseases may be linked to the immune system's capacity to manage stress. Orbai highlights that this area is currently under extensive investigation. "At what point does the stress on your body surpass your immune system's capability to cope? Understanding this could be pivotal in preventing autoimmune diseases before they manifest."

Nevertheless, Orbai points out that this hypothesis remains unverified, as numerous genetic and environmental factors influence autoimmunity. Researchers have yet to provide a conclusive explanation for the higher prevalence of these diseases in women compared to men.

The Role of Cortisol in Stress and Immunity

Brianna Chu (2022) adds that cortisol is a steroid hormone synthesised by the two adrenal glands located atop each kidney. In response to stress, the body releases increased levels of cortisol into the bloodstream. Maintaining an appropriate balance of cortisol is crucial for overall health, as both excessive and insufficient production can lead to various health issues. Excess cortisol impacts the immune system and is linked to mental disorders, pain, and disease.

Commonly referred to as the "stress hormone," cortisol plays numerous vital roles beyond merely managing the body's stress response.

It is also essential to recognise that there are several types of stress from a biological perspective, including trauma, acute stress, and chronic stress. During stressful situations, the body may release cortisol following the secretion of "fight or flight" hormones, such as adrenaline, to maintain a heightened state of alertness. Furthermore, cortisol facilitates the release of glucose from the liver, providing quick energy during stressful periods.

Environmental stress refers to the strain experienced due to unfavourable or challenging circumstances in the environment. Such conditions may include excessive noise, pollution, overcrowding, or hazardous living situations. These stressors can negatively impact both physical and mental well-being, leading to feelings of discomfort or anxiety. The body employs a complex system to regulate cortisol levels.

The hypothalamus, a small region of the brain responsible for hormonal control, along with the pituitary gland, a minute gland situated beneath the brain, governs cortisol production in the adrenal glands. When blood cortisol levels decrease, the hypothalamus secretes corticotropin-releasing hormone (CRH), prompting the pituitary gland to produce adrenocorticotropic hormone (ACTH). Subsequently, ACTH stimulates the adrenal glands to generate and release cortisol.

For optimal cortisol levels in the body, it is imperative that the hypothalamus, pituitary gland, and adrenal glands function effectively.

Chronic Inflammation and Disease

Chronic inflammation has been linked to an elevated risk of numerous diseases, such as infectious diseases, cardiovascular conditions, diabetes, certain types of cancer, and autoimmune disorders. One potential explanation for the connection between chronic stress and inflammation is the emergence of glucocorticoid receptor resistance resulting from prolonged exposure to stressors. This resistance can lead to the dysregulation of the hypothalamic-pituitary-adrenal (HPA) axis, which in turn affects inflammatory processes.

Deliana Infante's (2019) research, conducted on animal models, has demonstrated that chronic inflammation can induce sickness and behaviours resembling depression in response to ongoing stress.

Stress has the potential to disrupt both cellular and humoral immune responses, thereby heightening vulnerability to infectious diseases like influenza. It is also linked to the reactivation of dormant viruses, such as herpes simplex virus (HSV) and Epstein-Barr virus (EBV), as well as altered T-cell responses to antiviral vaccinations.

Moreover, acute psychological stress can trigger swift alterations in leukocyte dynamics, which may impact the body's ability to respond to autoimmune and viral threats.

The relationship between emotions and vulnerability to infections is bidirectional. A notable example of this connection is sepsis, which is defined by an unregulated immune response to severe infections and can lead to enduring psychiatric disorders, such as chronic anxiety and post-traumatic stress disorder.

Meta-analyses provide a historical overview of this area of study, consolidating knowledge acquired about the link between stress and human immunity since its initial investigation in the 1960s. This review emphasises recent and important discoveries regarding the stress-immune relationship in humans, including the immunological impacts of stress at various life stages, the mediators involved in the stress-immunity connection, environmental perspectives, and how this relationship is expressed in clinical populations.

The Overlooked Impact of Environmental Factors

Stress often originates physically, mentally, and emotionally in childhood and persists through various stages of life, including schools, media, and the workplace. It is exacerbated by exposure to pesticides, nutritional deficiencies, paint, carpet cleaning products, metal fillings, mercury, seafood, and mould.

Often, we overlook the obvious. If we apply pesticides to our food, which not only eradicates natural organisms but also degrades the soil, what impact do we expect it to have on our own health? We are, after all, a part of nature.

The cocktail Affect

There is a compilation of the most contaminated fruits and vegetables revealed in data provided by the UK Government, which indicates the percentage of samples that contain residues of multiple pesticides. Emphasis has been placed on recognising multiple residues due to the fact that our regulatory framework evaluates the safety of individual pesticides in isolation, neglecting the increasing evidence that the combination of chemicals can enhance their harmful effects.

This issue, referred to as the "cocktail effect," has been acknowledged as a significant concern both in the UK and internationally. Nevertheless, there has been insufficient action taken to comprehend or mitigate the potential health risks associated with prolonged exposure to mixtures of pesticides.

While the focus is often on fruits and vegetables in the context of the Dirty Dozen, various foods, including grains such as barley, oats, and wheat (and consequently bread), are also found to contain mixtures of pesticide residues.

According to government testing results from 2021, the percentage of bread products containing two or more pesticides nearly doubled from the previous year, reaching 50%. This represents a significant increase compared to the average of approximately 25% over the past decade. The tested bread products included standard white and brown bread, crumpets, scones, and muffins. A total of eleven different pesticides were identified, five of which are associated with cancer risk: cypermethrin, deltamethrin, flonicamid (insecticides), fosetyl (fungicide), and glyphosate (herbicide).

The presence of glyphosate in grains is primarily attributed to its application as a pre-harvest desiccant, used to artificially dry crops to facilitate harvesting. If the UK Government were to prohibit the use of glyphosate in this capacity, it could potentially decrease the levels of this residue found in grains.

In addition, pesticide residues in wine have become a significant concern. The results from the government's testing programme in 2022 revealed a substantial rise in the percentage of wine containing multiple pesticide residues, increasing from 14% in 2016 to 50% in 2022. The analysis of 72 wine samples identified residues of 19 different pesticides, an increase from 16 in 2016, including nine substances associated with cancer.

Glyphosate (herbicide) has been detected on apples. Concern regarding the health implications of glyphosate has been rising for several years. As the most commonly utilised herbicide, it has been linked to numerous health issues, including various cancers, birth defects, and kidney ailments. The demand for a prohibition on glyphosate has grown stronger, with several nations already banning its use or actively working towards its elimination. This chemical is not only employed in agricultural practices but is also extensively used in urban areas across the UK to manage weed growth.

The excessive use of pesticides in wine production not only endangers the health of British consumers but also affects individuals residing and working in wine-producing regions. Research conducted in France and published in October 2023 indicated that children living near densely planted vineyards face a heightened risk of developing leukaemia. Similarly, a study from Canada in 2006 highlighted that workers in the wine industry are at an increased risk of illnesses due to exposure to elevated pesticide levels in vineyards.

"Wine enthusiasts should not have to face the risk of exposure to a variety of harmful pesticides when enjoying a drink. The organic wine industry is thriving, demonstrating that it is entirely feasible to produce wine without the use of toxic chemicals," stated Nick Mole, Policy Officer at PAN UK.

Chlorpyrifos, an insecticide, has recently been banned for use within the EU; however, it remains as a residue on produce imported into the UK. Numerous epidemiological studies have linked chlorpyrifos exposure during pregnancy or childhood to lower birth weights and neurological alterations, including delayed motor development and attention difficulties. Furthermore, exposure to low levels of chlorpyrifos is increasingly correlated with changes in cognitive and behavioural performance in children. Chlorpyrifos is also suspected of being an endocrine disruptor.

One of the regularly detected pesticides is difenoconazole. This pesticide is employed to manage various issues, such as blight and seed rot. It is commonly found as a residue on most items listed in the Dirty Dozen. Numerous fungicides belonging to the 'azole' category, including this one, are believed to be endocrine-disrupting chemicals (EDCs). Additionally, difenoconazole is considered a potential human carcinogen and a reproductive or developmental toxin, which implies that it may negatively impact sexual health and fertility, diminish both the quantity and quality of sperm, and lead to miscarriages.

Lost in translation.

The egoic mind tends to complicate matters, adding things, changing the nature of things, or removing their essence.

Let's say that your vehicle ends up in a garage because you put diesel in it, but your vehicle takes petrol. The mechanic at the garage might say (tongue in cheek), "Oh dear, you've put the wrong liquid in the fuel tank." You ask, "Can you put a tablet in that will clean the fuel tank so I can add the petrol?" The mechanic replies, "No, that will not work!" (with a mind-boggling expression on their face).

They explain that the diesel must be removed, the tank and pipes cleaned, and only then can petrol be added.

The mechanic may not have a PhD, doctorate, or master's degree. They are dealing with a machine, and what is clear makes sense. The mechanic is trained to understand what the machine needs—no complication. It simply feels logical.

However, can you see why someone might ask if a pill can be added? This is the norm for the majority of society when it comes to a living body. After putting in the wrong fuel, the response is not just, "Yes," but rather, "You've come to the right place to add things in and remove things that don't work properly." We have been conditioned to take better care of objects than the most precious machine we will ever own—our bodies.

Although some scientists and doctors have stated that modern diseases disrupt the microbiome, the meaning of this statement can often be misinterpreted. It may suggest that the disease itself is responsible rather than the development of additives, food modifications, and pesticides sprayed on crops.

Food and the pesticides applied to it are subjects of considerable debate among professionals. It is surprising to observe that hospitals often stock unhealthy beverages and processed foods. Organic food options and healthier water alternatives, free from fluoride, appear to be absent. In contrast, animals exist without labels, educational institutions, or societal pressures regarding performance.

They are not subjected to the anxieties of consumer behaviour during crises, such as panic buying during a pandemic. Animals instinctively know what and when to eat, thriving in harmony with nature. The only species that exhibit illnesses akin to human conditions are domesticated or laboratory animals, as they are exposed to the same harmful products as we are.

Historical narratives do not necessarily reflect truth; often, they are distorted by ego and societal conditioning. The notion of being civilised or educated does not inherently equate to being correct or virtuous. Indoctrination leads individuals to adopt external beliefs, and the longer one is subjected to it, the more likely they are to conform. In quantum physics, we discover that our perceptions shape our reality, influenced by the beliefs of those from whom we learn.

Is Science Correct?

Science, by definition, is the pursuit and application of knowledge and understanding of the natural and social world through a systematic methodology based on evidence.

Many individuals regard science with a reverence akin to that of a sacred deity. It is frequently stated that science has made significant discoveries. However, as this book suggests, much of what we accept as truth is founded on falsehoods. Science is often subject to revision—or more accurately, the beliefs of individuals who once held a particular view only to later realise their error.

My perspective on science as a deception stems from the understanding that we are creators of our own realities, encompassing both positive and negative experiences. A substantial portion of our beliefs originates from falsehoods perpetuated by previous generations. Taught these inaccuracies at home or in educational settings, they have passed them down. Furthermore, we are contributing to our own detriment and that of the planet, all in the name of scientific pursuits and dogmatic beliefs that lack truth.

For instance, a client attended her regular appointment while experiencing a cold. She apologised, saying, "I always catch a cold at this time of year." I responded, "So, by believing that, you have effectively invited the cold to return next year?"

Science appears to be something used to validate a belief that must be manipulated for our benefit. From my discoveries, this can often be detrimental. This is because humans possess the ego.

What are we educated with?

Part of my point is captured in this quote: *"Give me the boy aged seven, and I will show you the man."* There is no clear agreement on who originally said it—some attribute it to Aristotle, while others link it to a Jesuit motto. This idea was later supported by Freud and Bowlby, a British psychiatrist and psychoanalyst, in their studies on child development and how early life experiences shape adulthood. Early doctrines not only remain but also replay through generations, manifesting in various forms, such as ideological "isms."

For instance, in my early experiences growing up in a so-called *civilised society*, I was often called names like "Niger" or "black bastard" and told to go back to my own country. I would have gladly gone back—if it had been possible—but I was born here, so I lived in the hellhole of this one.

However, even as a child, I understood that no country truly belongs to any of us because this planet is not of our creation. The hell I experienced was not the land itself but the projections of the minds that surrounded me.

The part of the world I grew up in was tough, and I had to adhere to the rules set by the dictators of my environment. These rules became second nature, especially during my school days at the age of seven.

One such moment occurred during P.E. class. We were playing on the gym equipment, setting up the climbing frame, which included ropes and rings. My favourite teacher at the time, Miss Bough, decided that we would end the session with a game of tag, which we called "Tig." I loved P.E. and was quite flexible and agile due to my gymnastics training. We all dashed around, trying to stay on the equipment—balancing on benches and swinging from the climbing frame—while the caretaker chased us.

I was enjoying myself until I realised that the popular Caucasian boy was the last one left after everyone else had either been caught or touched the ground. I noticed a glance exchanged between Miss Bough and the caretaker, who nodded in agreement, and I instinctively understood: the favourite boy would not be tagged. Instead, the caretaker would focus on catching me.

Eventually, I stopped dodging and walked over to him, extending my arm so he could tag me. It dawned on me then—there were unspoken rules at play in this game. The expressions on both the caretaker's and the favourite boy's faces mirrored each other, and I wondered if mine looked the same.

We were all participating in a performance shaped by societal expectations. The favourite boy was declared the winner, but the look exchanged between us suggested that we all knew it was not a fair victory.

We were trapped in a falsehood—even those who recognised the truth but were too afraid to acknowledge it. From that moment on, I lost trust in Miss Bough. I began to see that even those with seemingly kind and caring names could be deceptive. Ironically, the school I attended was called *All Saints.*

Moving the Spotlight

For centuries, humanity has subjected the human body to blame, accusation, punishment, rape, murder, and colonisation. The concept of *moving the spotlight* refers to the act of the perpetrator shifting blame onto the victim through deceit. Numerous narratives throughout history—and in modern-day society—exemplify this phenomenon.

Although the truth may often be apparent, people frequently become complacent or selectively acknowledge only the information that aligns with their ego-driven narratives. They accept the first available explanation or the one that provides the most comfort.

How often have you held a belief about an individual or a group, only to later discover that your assumption was unfounded? When you reflect on your emotions, do you ever feel guilt? If so, do you respond with anger, defensiveness, or deflection—evading accountability and creating internal dissonance?

Conversely, when you are innocent, you may feel curiosity, hurt, and perplexity. You maintain a sense of internal harmony even when facing external discord.

How many people do you instinctively know you can be honest with, and how many do you hesitate to speak openly with out of fear of consequences?

The Dogon tribe of West Africa has long possessed advanced astronomical knowledge, suggesting that ancient civilisations had profound insights about the universe and themselves—knowledge that was not derived from human sources. This information is documented in writings attributed to the god Thoth.

While society often promotes the notion that humans are the pinnacle of intelligence, contemporary realities suggest otherwise.

They reveal a pervasive state of mental distress and a culture steeped in harmful practices, both physically and emotionally.

Throughout history, we have been taught that slaves built the pyramids. However, it makes more sense that they were constructed using advanced technology that harnessed the Earth's energy and sound vibrations—technology that humans did not possess.

History indicates that the transatlantic slave trade began in 1444, when the first cargo of human slaves was captured and brought to Lisbon, Portugal. However, the Western European slave market was initially composed of people from Europe.

Roman Slavery

Roman slaves were typically individuals captured in battle and taken to Rome to be sold. In addition to this, abandoned children could also be raised as slaves. According to Roman law, fathers had the authority to sell their older children if they were facing financial difficulties.

Wealthy Romans purchased slaves at marketplaces, with young male slaves who possessed a skill fetching the highest prices, as they could work for many years. Once purchased, a slave remained a slave for life unless granted freedom by their owner or if they managed to buy their own freedom.

However, buying one's freedom required raising the same amount of money that had been paid for them—often an impossible task. If a slave married and had children, their offspring automatically became slaves as well.

British Captives on the Barbary Coast

Pirates known as Barbary pirates, or Ottoman Corsairs, were active in North Africa (referred to as the *Barbary Coast*). They operated from Tunis, Tripoli, Algiers, and various ports in Morocco, targeting ships in the western Mediterranean Sea from the era of the Crusades to the early 19th century.

These pirates also raided ships travelling to Asia via Africa and even attacked coastal towns from the Adriatic to Ireland and Iceland. During the late 1500s and early 1600s, it was estimated that approximately 35,000 European Christian captives were held as slaves on the Barbary Coast. The majority were sailors captured along with their vessels, while others included fishermen and residents of coastal villages.

These white slaves were typically from impoverished backgrounds and had little chance of regaining their freedom—much like the Africans enslaved in America. Many spent their lives in servitude, succumbing to starvation, illness, or abuse. Slaves were often resold multiple times, with the most unfortunate abandoned in the desert or forced to row in the Turkish sultan's galleys for years without ever setting foot on land.

Numerous Dutch, German, and British captives remained in captivity for extended periods, lacking assistance from structured religious institutions or government resources to secure their release. Those enslaved in Barbary came from diverse backgrounds, encompassing various races and religions, including black, brown, white, Catholic, Protestant, Orthodox, Jewish, and Muslim. In this context, there was no discrimination based on colour or faith.

The individuals who were enslaved or imprisoned had the possibility of being ransomed. For instance, Queen Elizabeth I sought to persuade the 'Negroes' living in Britain to voluntarily surrender themselves to a trader named Caspar Van Senden. This trader from Lübeck informed the Queen that he could sell them as slaves in Spain and Portugal, which would allow her to recover his costs associated with ransoming and returning some English prisoners held in those regions.

It appears that neither the free Africans nor the proprietors of enslaved Africans in Britain were willing to comply with the Queen's decree, prompting her to issue it multiple times.

Stamped from the Beginning

The documentary *Stamped from the Beginning* tells the truth about slavery and racism. One reason I say it tells the truth is that, based on what was historically claimed, I would not have been capable of writing this book—simply because of the colour of my skin, which supposedly meant I was of low intellect.

In the 1860s, Senator Jefferson Davis of Mississippi opposed a bill funding education for black people. Davis justified his opposition by fabricating a story about black inferiority. He claimed that he had found information in the Bible stating that Cain had been exiled from the Garden of Eden.

According to his story, Cain came across a land called Nod, where creatures existed before Adam and Eve. These creatures, he alleged, were black people—beasts and inferior to white people. Davis stated that black inferiority was the will of God.

This fabricated narrative gave free rein to the British to pillage, rape, torture, starve, and imprison children, men, and women. It justified the theft of land, minerals, gold, and silver from Africa, all under the guise of divine will.

Europeans were unable to deploy armies to conquer or abduct Africans; instead, they were compelled to acquire individuals through transactions with local kings and chiefs. Traders employed various strategies to incite warfare, as Africans were generally inclined to sell only prisoners of war.

The allure of European commodities, particularly firearms and ammunition, ultimately led to the emergence of kidnapping gangs that targeted neighbouring communities. Those who were captured or taken prisoner were forced to march to the coast, where they awaited sale. The number of individuals who perished during these raids, conflicts, and forced marches remains uncertain. It is possible that the fatalities could rival the number of those ultimately transported, which is estimated to be between 12 and 20 million.

It is important to highlight that the African sellers were unaware of the horrific forms of slavery that Europeans implemented in their colonies.

Africans actively resisted abduction and fought against those attempting to capture them in warfare. However, their lack of access to firearms severely diminished their chances of success. Moreover, the further one resided from the coast, the less likely they were to possess firearms.

The relentless violence and kidnappings, coupled with the centuries-long exportation of millions of the most capable and vigorous members of the population, have undoubtedly had enduring effects that persist to this day.

The majority of slaves were not directly transported to Britain, with only a few thousand making the journey there. Instead, they were taken to British colonies in the Caribbean and various nations in America. Approximately 3 million slaves were transported from Africa by the British, while an additional 9 million were transported by other nations.

Certain regions experienced significant advantages due to Britain's participation in the slave trade. Areas that accumulated the greatest wealth from slavery observed total income surges exceeding 40%, alongside a population growth of 6.5%. Additionally, the income of capitalists more than doubled, while the earnings of landlords saw a slight decrease of just over 7%.

The Superiority Complexes

Some of the experiences of slaves came at the hands of those who named themselves the superior, intelligent, genteel, gentry, or civilised people—those who were bowed down to in the splendour of their spoils from the enslavement of human beings. This behaviour is likened to the doctrine of Adolf Hitler, who came into conflict with Britain and other countries.

The First World War and the subsequent peace agreements led to the emergence of new aspirations, rivalries, and tensions. There was widespread hope that the post-war peace arrangements would establish a new global order and prevent the recurrence of the devastation witnessed during the war.

The Treaty of Versailles, signed in June 1919, established the League of Nations—an international organisation aimed at fostering peace and averting conflict. Nevertheless, the treaty represented a risky compromise, as each of the victorious Allies—Britain, the United States, France, and Italy—sought to advance their own national interests. Germany was compelled to cede territory, disarm, and compensate for the damages incurred during the war.

Many in Britain and America criticised these punitive measures as excessively harsh. The stipulations of the treaty incited immediate outrage and enduring resentment within Germany.

The feelings of defeat, humiliation, and perceived injustice significantly influenced both German foreign and domestic policies, with demands for a revision of the treaty's terms becoming a prominent issue in international relations during the 1920s and 1930s. The interwar period was characterised by instability and insecurity, exacerbated by the collapse of the global economy in 1929.

Hitler was the dictator of Nazi Germany for 12 years. During his reign, he believed his work was providence and often invoked God in his speeches, referring to "the God who let iron grow." Nazi Germany perpetrated mass murder on an unparalleled scale. The Nazis, along with their allies and collaborators, were responsible for the deaths of six million Jewish individuals.

This organised, state-sanctioned genocide is referred to as the Holocaust. Additionally, the Nazis and their associates committed numerous other mass atrocities, targeting and exterminating millions of non-Jewish individuals during World War II.

The British Empire constituted a global network of territories governed or managed by the United Kingdom and its predecessor states for nearly four centuries, commencing in the late 1500s. This empire encompassed colonies across America, Africa, Asia, and Australasia. At its zenith, it governed over 400 million individuals. Recognised as the largest empire in history, the British Empire emerged as a significant global power for a century.

The motivations behind the establishment of the empire included the pursuit of wealth, the acquisition of power, and the dissemination of Christianity alongside British cultural practices.

The empire experienced a significant loss of some of its oldest and most overcrowded North American colonies following the American War of Independence in 1783.

During World War II, Japan seized control of Britain's territories in East and Southeast Asia. The post-war period marked the onset of decolonisation, ultimately leading to the decline of the empire.

Slavery persisted for approximately 300 years, though records continue to document its presence even today.

"Dieu et mon droit" is a phrase in French that translates to "God and my right." This motto is associated with the British royal family and is featured on the coat of arms of the United Kingdom. It is believed that King Henry V first adopted this motto in the 15th century, signifying the divine right of the monarch to rule.

An article written by the historian Brooke Newman was published in *The Guardian* on 6 April 2023. Newman describes how, from the archives of slavery, it is evident that the voices of those who were enslaved are rarely heard and have been systematically excluded.

The article:

On 27 March 2007, nearly 450 years after Elizabeth I sponsored John Hawkins' slaving expeditions to west Africa, Elizabeth II attended a service in Westminster Abbey to commemorate the bicentenary of Britain's abolition of the slave trade. Rowan

Williams, the archbishop of Canterbury, delivered a sermon focused on slavery's "hideously persistent" legacies. "We, who are the heirs of the slave-owning and slave-trading nations of the past, have to face the fact that our historic prosperity was built in large part on this atrocity," he said.

Moments later a Black protester dashed in front of the altar, disrupting the service with shouts of "This is an insult to us!" Her face impassive, Queen Elizabeth watched as security guards struggled with the protester, Toyin Agbetu, founder of the pan-African human rights organisation Ligali. As he was forcibly ejected, Agbetu pointed at the queen and yelled: "You, the queen, should be ashamed! You should say sorry!" In keeping with her own protocol and that of her namesake, Elizabeth I, whose motto was video et taceo (I see and keep silent), Queen Elizabeth said nothing.

"The voice of our complaint," the Black abolitionist Ottobah Cugoano warned the British public and George III in Thoughts and sentiments on the evil of slavery (1787), "ought to sound in your ears as the rolling waves around your circum-ambient shores; and if it is not harkened unto, it may yet arise with a louder voice, as the rolling thunder." Mary Prince, the first Black woman to publish an account of her enslavement in Britain in 1831, agreed to share her harrowing life story to ensure "that good people in England might hear from a slave what a slave had felt and suffered".

It's rare for Britons, both then and now, to hear the voices of enslaved people. The transatlantic slave system that commodified its captives, transforming Africans and their descendants into human chattel, was not designed to preserve their experiences or perspectives. Its sole purpose was to generate profit for its operators. As the Kittitian-British novelist Caryl Phillips put it in The Atlantic Sound: "You were transported in a wooden vessel across a broad expanse of water to a place which rendered your tongue silent."

That compulsory silence extends to the archive of slavery. Although archives are full of stories, the voices they preserve are limited, fragmentary and far from neutral. They are, in most cases, the voices of enslavers, who continue to impart their outlook and version of events to future readers. "In history," the Haitian scholar Michel-Rolph Trouillot observed, "power begins at the source."

It begins in the surviving ledgers, ship manifests and stock books of slave-trading companies, in plantation account books 191ataloguing births and deaths, and in the bound volumes of state correspondence between British officials and colonial administrators that line the shelves of archives. Through these manuscript materials, historians are granted access to the institutional records of the Atlantic slave system. But rarely to the enslaved themselves.

The dehumanising horrors of slavery are replicated in the archive. "The objectification of the enslaved allowed authorities to reduce them to valued objects to be bought and sold, used to produce profit and to retain and bequeath wealth," the historian Marisa

Fuentes has argued. "This same objectification led to the violence in and of the archive." The reduction of African people to commodities can be seen in the archival document I shared with the Guardian showing the 1689 transfer of £1,000 of shares in the slave-trading Royal African Company to King William III from Edward Colston, the company's deputy governor.

To do justice to their subjects, historians of slavery must grapple with the problematic nature of the archive. However, the limitations of the archive do not explain why, as the coronation of Charles III nears, the British monarchy has not apologised for its historic links to slavery. The paper trail of crown involvement in slavery, though incomplete, is nonetheless extensive. As Saidiya Hartman noted in Lose Your Mother: "Money multiplied if fed human blood." That British monarchs and members of the royal family invested in and profited from the slave trade and Atlantic slavery is indisputable.

Still, if we hear anything about Britain's or the British crown's role in the enslavement and death of millions of Africans, the focus is almost always on abolition, not slavery. This deliberate rewriting of history, this purposeful forgetting, echoes a triumphalist narrative of national progress initiated more than 200 years ago by the famed abolitionist Thomas Clarkson. Popular support for abolition, he reflected in 1808, "overpowered me with joy. I rejoiced in it because it was a proof of the general good disposition of my countrymen."

Passing legislation to abolish the slave trade in 1807 and then slavery itself in 1833 (after a period of forced "apprenticeship"), decades before the hard-fought victory of emancipation in the US, reshaped Britain's collective memory. Its central role, and that of the monarchy's, in the expansion of the transatlantic slave trade and horrors of Atlantic slavery was overwritten, replaced by a celebratory national history focused on the Christian conviction of Britain's white abolitionist campaigners.

The Colston connection: how Prince William's Kensington Palace home is linked to slavery.

Since 1807, Britain has told itself and the world that it is an abolitionist nation. An abolitionist nation that rejected human bondage, championing the rights of formerly enslaved people and their descendants as equal subjects of the crown. According to this national narrative, though slavery, in the words of Prince Albert in 1840, represented "the blackest stain on civilised Europe", it was Britain that led the way toward its eradication.

But this version of British history is nothing but a muddled, self-congratulatory national myth, one no less misleading and historically dubious than the myth of American exceptionalism. The history of Atlantic slavery is equally a British story and an American story. They are separate yet interdependent strands of the same sordid tale; we cannot fully understand one without the other.

"Those of us living in the rich societies of the west have all, albeit profoundly unequally, enjoyed the fruits of racial capitalism,"

stressed historian Catherine Hall, head of UCL's Legacies of British Slavery project; "we are all survivors of slavery, not just those who can directly trace their lineages."

Evidence of royal involvement in what the UN has labelled "the greatest crime against humanity" committed in the modern era saturates the archive of slavery. King Charles has for the first time signalled his support for research into the monarchy's historical links with transatlantic slavery. But more should be done to listen and respond to the descendants of the enslaved.

A nation's culture is shaped by its shared history, collective experiences, and the self-perception held by its citizens. This foundation influences the behaviours, customs, beliefs, and attitudes prevalent among the populace. Nunn emphasises the crucial role of history in cultural formation, as it is referenced to establish concepts of national heritage and tradition.

Between the 16th and 19th centuries, the British military, including its Army, served as an instrument of the British Empire, facilitating the transatlantic slave trade. Rooted in a white-supremacist ideology that deemed black Africans inferior to their white European counterparts, this system forcibly removed black Africans, subjecting them to slave labour in Britain's Caribbean colonies.

The transatlantic slave trade functioned as a British institution for 245 years, from 1562 to 1807, meaning its abolition occurred more recently than its duration. The enduring legacy of this trade continues to impact society today. British institutions and society flourished under a structural framework that exploited black Africans for the advantage of white British citizens, who benefited from the labour of enslaved individuals while remaining largely oblivious to the horrific nature of the practice.

As Eddo-Lodge points out, the emancipation of enslaved individuals in 1838 did not lead to an immediate transformation in societal attitudes towards black colonial subjects. Many in the predominantly white British public continued to regard black colonial subjects as inferior, and these individuals navigated their newfound freedom within a context of pervasive racism.

The onset of the First World War in 1914 marked the advent of large-scale warfare across various continents. This necessitated the extensive mobilisation of subjects from the British Empire to enlist in military service, which included the formation of regiments from British colonies in the Caribbean. Seventy-six years after the abolition of slavery, this situation arguably provided the British Army with its first significant opportunity to incorporate black soldiers into its ranks.

Nevertheless, the experiences of black soldiers were not comparable to those of their white peers. Black units were prohibited from engaging in combat alongside or against white Europeans on the Western Front; those black soldiers who enlisted as infantrymen were often relegated to labour battalions during their deployment in Europe. The British Government was concerned that permitting black soldiers to "fight alongside whites and against whites" would undermine the entire colonial hierarchy, which was fundamentally rooted in white supremacy.

Imperial War Museums records indicate that, less than a year after the end of the First World War, no black units were invited to participate in the 1919 victory parade at the Cenotaph in London. This exclusion was part of a calculated effort by the British Government to minimise the recognition of black soldiers' contributions, thereby reinforcing a predominantly white European perspective of the First World War among the British public—a viewpoint that persists to this day.

The King elucidates how the lack of acknowledgement for the contributions of black soldiers has sustained the notion of the British Army as being primarily Anglo-Saxon in its identity. Furthermore, there is scant evidence to suggest any cultural shift during the interwar years. By 1938, policies still barred the integration of black soldiers into the British Army, as Army Order 89 limited recruitment to individuals of "pure European descent," highlighting the ongoing presence of racism and discrimination within the military (Steve, 2024).

Despite the lack of recognition, Walter Tull has emerged as the most renowned black British soldier of the First World War. He enlisted in December 1914, experienced shell shock, and subsequently returned to combat during the Battle of the Somme, earning the 1914-15 Star along with various British war and victory medals.

In 1917, he was commissioned as an officer and was recognised in dispatches for his "gallantry and coolness" during the Battle of Piave in Italy in January 1918. Tragically, just two months later, he lost his life in No Man's Land during the Second Battle of the Somme. Following his passing, his superiors communicated with his family to inform them that he had been nominated for a Military Cross. However, this nomination was declined without any justification, suggesting that the refusal was influenced by his race. Vasili articulates that Tull "ridiculed the strongly entrenched belief of the Army Council that white enlisted personnel would not accept commands from a black individual."

As the centenary of the First World War was commemorated from 2014 to 2018, it is important to recognise that many individuals have been overlooked in historical accounts and deserve acknowledgment.

Following Britain's entry into the First World War on 4 August 1914, black recruits were present across all branches of the military. From the onset of the conflict, black Britons volunteered at recruitment centres, joined by West Indian colonials who travelled from the Caribbean to the "Mother Country" at their own expense to contribute to the fight against Germany. Their assistance was crucial, and they provided it willingly.

Shortly after the war commenced, soldiers from Nigeria, the Gold Coast, Sierra Leone, Gambia, and other African colonies were enlisted. They played a vital role in defending their nations' borders adjacent to German territories and later significantly contributed to the efforts to expel German forces from Africa. Throughout the conflict, 60,000 black South Africans and 120,000 other Africans served in uniformed labour units.

Among the most devoted to his King and country was Lionel Turpin, a Guyanese merchant seaman. At just 19 years of age, he enlisted in the British Army and was deployed with No. 32 British Expeditionary Force to the Western Front in Europe. He participated in the battles of the Somme, and his military service concluded in 1919, marked by the receipt of two medals, the lasting effects of gas exposure, and a shell wound in his back.

Lionel passed away in 1929 due to the lingering effects of gas exposure during the war. His experience reflects the broader narrative of numerous black colonials who supported the "Mother Country" during the First World War.

In 1915, a decision was made to establish a distinct West Indian contingent to contribute to the war effort. This led to the formation of the British West Indies Regiment (BWIR), a separate unit comprised of black soldiers within the British Army.

The initial recruits departed from Jamaica and arrived in Britain in October 1915, where they underwent training at a camp located near Seaford on the Sussex coast. By the conclusion of the war in

November 1918, a total of 15,204 black men had served in the BWIR.

Despite their service, the black soldiers of the BWIR were predominantly commanded by white officers and were primarily assigned non-combat roles in regions such as Egypt, Mesopotamia, and parts of Europe. For instance, in July 1916, the 3rd and 4th battalions of the BWIR were dispatched to France and Belgium to perform duties as ammunition carriers.

The BWIR engaged in various labour-intensive tasks, including loading ammunition, laying telephone lines, and digging trenches, yet they were not authorised to engage in combat as a battalion. By the war's end, the BWIR had suffered the loss of 185 soldiers, either killed in action or succumbing to their wounds. Additionally, 1,071 men died from illness, and 697 were injured.

Seaford Cemetery is the final resting place for over 300 Commonwealth war graves, with nineteen headstones bearing the crest of the BWIR. While some black servicemen made the ultimate sacrifice, the contributions of these individuals have largely been overlooked over time, with the notable exception of Walter Tull (Black History 365, n.d.; Steve, 2024).

More recently, Indian historian Vijay Prashad addressed the issue of white supremacy at a conference in Glasgow, where he began by praising the city's beauty. However, this admiration prompted him to reflect on the implications of such beautiful cities in the West. He referenced a poignant observation by Walter

Benjamin, the German-Jewish philosopher, who noted that every monument of civilisation also serves as a monument of barbarism.

This reflection led Prashad to discuss the famine in Bengal, highlighting the plight of jute workers who sent their produce to Dundee via Glasgow's ports, as well as the enslaved Africans transported from Ghana to the New World, all of which contributed to the wealth of the UK, particularly London and Glasgow.

Between 1765 and 1938, the British Isles appropriated £45 trillion from India. When India expelled the British, its literacy rate stood at a mere 13%. The exploitation extended to natural resources, exemplified by the Jharia coal mine in Jharkhand, which has been burning underground since at least 1916.

This ongoing disaster has resulted in the loss of 37 million tonnes of coal and rendered 220 billion tonnes inaccessible, while also causing ground instability, structural damage, and respiratory illnesses. The underground fires in the Jharia coal mine represent a significant environmental crisis with far-reaching negative effects.

Prashad expressed his discontent with the condescending attitudes of politicians such as Boris Johnson, Joe Biden, and Emmanuel Macron, which have persisted for centuries and remain evident today. He argued that colonialism is not merely a historical phenomenon but a continuous condition, reflected in the mindset that perpetuates blame on the colonised while ignoring the underlying greed and barbarism of nations like the United States and the UK.

These countries continue to exploit resources by outsourcing production to nations like China, only to shift the blame for pollution onto them. Furthermore, Prashad criticised the practice of lending money to India that rightfully belongs to India, stating, "You give us our money back as debt, then you lecture us on how we should live."

These are the colonial institutions that perpetuate themselves year after year. The climate justice movement expresses concern for the future; however, Prashad questions, "What future?" He points out that children in Asia, Africa, and Latin America lack a present, let alone a future.

The prevailing slogan emphasises worry about the future, yet Prashad urges a focus on the current situation. He characterises this concern as a "middle-class bourgeois Western slogan." Prashad underscores the fact that 2.7 billion individuals are experiencing hunger while the West advocates for reduced consumption. He concludes by asking whether those in the West are prepared to acknowledge the actions of their politicians, which have been driven by business interests and greed.

(Prashad, 2024).

"You think your pain and your heartbreak are unprecedented in the history of the world, but then you read. It was books that taught me that the things that tormented me most were the very things that connected me with all the people who were alive, who had ever been alive."

James Baldwin

Freedom To Speak the truth?

Malcolm X's advocacy in the 1960s is now being acknowledged as society begins to recognise its own subjugation. There are frequent calls for a return to a so-called greatness in Britain, prompting the question: for whom was it truly great, and whom does it serve?

The remnants of the slave trade persist, albeit in a form that appears slightly more impartial. Malcolm X asserted that the black man is a puppet of the white man; however, I contend that we are all puppets, labouring for those who have thrived through our indoctrination and deception for their own gain. This dynamic has been a constant throughout history.

We possess the capacity to liberate ourselves. Jeshua/Jesus proclaimed, "The truth will set you free." Yet, as Jack Nicholson famously remarked in the film *A Few Good Men*, "The truth? You can't handle the truth."

What I mean by this is that, to my understanding, my creator has given all of us a conscience—a moral sense of right and wrong. My feelings, my awareness of something being wrong in the world, and what is written in plain sight affirm this truth.

We are now all equal slaves. We have been taught in the prison of school to learn through commands such as *must, should, have to,* and *got to.* We have been programmed to comply, obey, and not ask questions. From a young age, our voices, views, and feelings have been suppressed. The greatest tool that keeps us in servitude is **fear**.

Fear has kept us from looking at information outside of the *cult'ure's* teachings. We **think** the way we have been programmed to think. We eat what we have been programmed to eat. We fear what we have been programmed to fear. Whom do we fear? The government and business owners—those who take what is rightfully ours.

You may have experienced injustices in school, such as dealing with a bully whom you feared, and yet no one truly did anything about it. You may have interpreted this as meaning you were "not good enough." You are then fed chemicals that make you sick and are subsequently given more chemicals to try to feel better. You are bombarded with negative psychological junk food—information you believe to be true but often is not.

By now, we are not merely victims of our circumstances but have become participants through wilful ignorance, believing and trusting in labels we have been taught are trustworthy. We often do not investigate further but instead follow our homogeneous group to maintain our narrative of comfort. We are intellectually lazy.

The truth, as I see it from my findings regarding legislation, revolves around conscience and the essence of being human—an energy that works in harmony with all creation. We are sovereign and autonomous, yet we have been born into a system that distorts its own foundations. This system does not serve to benefit humankind but to govern over us, whether knowingly or unknowingly.

We have been so conditioned to do as we are told and taught to serve those whom we believe work in our best interests. However, it is those in positions of power who control us. But does that mean they truly have authority over us? If they did, we would not need to be conditioned from school to obey without question, nor would we need the constant insertion of fear through the threat of consequences.

The law of conscience was written, yet this seems to have been lost in translation—just as many other truths have been omitted from our education system. This system has been shaped by those deemed as leaders or, more accurately, enslavers.

From the moment we enter education until the day we leave, we are subjected to control. Those who govern over us have taken charge of our water, food, medicine, homes, liberty, freedom, transportation, land, and even the sky.

We are often told that our laws are outdated and must be replaced by those who rule over us. But who truly benefits from these changes?

Our Rights in Plain Sight.

Here is an example of some of our human rights, but I see a big disparity between what is written versus what I have experienced throughout my life—and still experience now—as well as what I witness others going through.

The concept of freedom of movement appears to be compromised, as I perceive it, due to the imposition of taxes and penalty fines associated with driving. When one navigates the Earth as a sovereign individual, this freedom is curtailed by mechanisms of force, fear, and authoritarianism, primarily serving the interests of others. These individuals, who share the same human dignity, are not above the law; however, financial exploitation persists, as highlighted in the Slavery Act.

Extortion

Extortion is defined in the Theft Act 1968 as: *"Making an unwarranted demand with menaces."*

Extortion refers to the unlawful use of intimidation to force someone to give up money, property, or services. We are commanded to hand over our money—or face being kidnapped (taken away), imprisoned (held captive), and having our human rights violated. The meaning of these words remains the same, yet we are led to believe that different rules apply to different people, as the saying goes: *different strokes for different folks.*

Modern Slavery Act 2015

Securing services, etc., by force, threats, or deception:

(5) The person is subjected to force, threats, or deception designed to induce him or her—

(a) To provide services of any kind.

(b) To provide another person with benefits of any kind.

(c) To enable another person to acquire benefits of any kindTypes of Coercive Control

Section 76 of the Serious Crime Act 2015 (SCA 2015) created the offence of controlling or coercive behaviour in an intimate or family relationship (CCB). It can be tried summarily or on indictment and carries a maximum penalty of five years' imprisonment.

Controlling behaviours may include:

- Isolating you from your family or friends.
- Controlling what you eat, wear, or do.
- Controlling who you are allowed to see or spend time with.
- Preventing you from accessing support.
- Gaslighting.
- Monitoring your behaviour (online or in person).
- Tracking you, for example, using your phone or car.
- Controlling your finances, including your ability to earn or spend money.

- Emotionally or physically threatening or intimidating you.

- Threatening to disclose personal information about you publicly.

- Humiliating or degrading you.

- Repeatedly putting you down.

- Making you feel fearful or scared of non-compliance.

Universal Declaration of Human Rights – UNITEDNATIONS (1948)

Now, therefore, The General Assembly proclaims this Universal Declaration of Human Rights

"As a common standard of achievement for all peoples and all nations, to the end that every individual and every organ of society, keeping this Declaration constantly in mind, shall strive by teaching and education to promote respect for these rights and freedoms and by progressive measures, national and international, to secure their universal and effective recognition and observance, both among the peoples of Member States themselves and among the peoples of territories under their jurisdiction.

All human beings are born free and equal in dignity and rights. They are endowed with reason and conscience and should act towards one another in a spirit of brotherhood.

Everyone is entitled to all the rights and freedoms set forth in this Declaration, without distinction of any kind, such as race, colour, sex, language, religion, political or other opinion, national or social origin, property, birth or other status.

Furthermore, no distinction shall be made on the basis of the political, jurisdictional or international status of the country or territory to which a person belongs, whether it be independent, trust, non-self-governing or under any other limitation of sovereignty.

Everyone is entitled to all the rights and without distinction of any kind, such as freedoms set forth in this Declaration, race, colour, sex, language, religion, political or other opinion, national or social origin, property, birth or other status. Furthermore, no distinction shall be made on the basis of the political, jurisdictional or international status of the country or territory to which a person belongs, whether it be independent, trust, non-self-governing or under any other limitation of sovereignty.

Everyone has the right to life, liberty and security of person. No one shall be held in slavery or servitude; slavery and the slave trade shall be prohibited in all their forms.

No one shall be subjected to torture or to cruel, inhuman or degrading treatment or punishment.

Everyone has the right to recognition everywhere as a person before the law.

All are equal before the law and are entitled without any discrimination to equal protection of the law. All are entitled to equal protection against any discrimination in violation of this Declaration and against any incitement to such discrimination.

Everyone has the right to an effective remedy by the competent national tribunals for acts violating the fundamental rights granted him by the constitution or by law.

No one shall be subjected to arbitrary arrest, detention or exile.

Everyone is entitled in full equality to a fair and public hearing by an independent and impartial tribunal, in the determination of his rights and obligations and of any criminal charge against him.

No one shall be subjected to arbitrary interference with his privacy, family, home or correspondence, nor to attacks upon his honour and reputation. Everyone has the right to the protection of the law against such interference or attacks.

Everyone has the right to freedom of movement and residence within the borders of each State.

Everyone has the right to leave any country, including his own, and to return to his country.

(1) Everyone has the right to own property alone as well as in association with others.

(2) No one shall be arbitrarily deprived of his property.

Everyone has the right to freedom of thought, conscience and religion; this right includes freedom to change his religion or belief, and freedom, either alone or in community with others and in public or private, to manifest his religion or belief in teaching, practice, worship and observance.

(1) Everyone has the right to take part in the government of his country, directly or through freely chosen representatives.

(2) Everyone has the right to equal access to public service in his country.

(3) The will of the people shall be the basis of the authority of government; this will shall be expressed in periodic and genuine elections which shall be by universal and equal suffrage and shall be held by secret vote or by equivalent free voting procedures.

Everyone, as a member of society, has to realization, through national the right to social security and is entitled effort and international cooperation and in accordance with the organization and resources of each State, of the economic, social and cultural rights indispensable for his dignity and the free development of his personality."

The Modern Slavery Act 2015, the Serious Crime Act 2015, and the Universal Declaration of Human Rights by the United Nations (1948) appear to be collectively violated. The predominant challenges we face from birth and throughout our lives stem from the very control from which we are meant to be liberated.

When a truth exists, it should apply universally; however, I have yet to witness the effective implementation of these acts in their entirety.

Human Rights.

Is it necessary for human science to intrude upon our essence, given that the creator of the apple also designed humanity to explore our fundamental nature?

Many cultures have pondered this question, leading one to consider whether science is merely appropriating age-old wisdom and presenting it as novel discoveries. Within each of us exists an innate voice that expresses discomfort, urging us to awaken and heed our own insights rather than conforming to external narratives.

Should educational institutions function merely as repetitive factories of narratives that define who we are not and how we should operate? Alternatively, ought they to serve as environments that foster an understanding of human nature and promote genuine learning about humanity?

The structure of our lives appears to be predetermined even before our birth. The language we speak, the clothing we wear, the environment in which we rest, the labels assigned to us, the food we consume, the individuals responsible for our education, and the cultural norms we adhere to all seem to be established without our consent. How can we claim to possess freedom when we have never been consulted, but rather instructed?

Women have fought for equal rights, yet this struggle has often resulted in separating parents from their children, placing their care in the hands of unfamiliar individuals. There exists a lack of genuine freedom of choice, as we are bound by an incessant obligation to conform to the demands to hand over not only our money, but ourselves and our offspring, which govern our lives. It is not the bills that are capped; it is our very existence that is limited, physically and financially.

The SOUL

The intangible nature of an individual refers to a non-physical component of a person that is thought to persist beyond death, encompassing their identity, character, and recollections. In various religious and philosophical frameworks, the soul is regarded as the spiritual element of a person that possesses the potential for salvation.

The great guru Bhagawan Ramana Maharshi stated that all creatures are an equal manifestation of the supreme self. Animals also elevate consciousness. Maharshi believed that every creature has the same rights as us. They were on Earth before us and have a right to their land; if they could speak our language, they would claim it.

It has become clear that the ego entangles us in stories that become increasingly complicated to unravel, as egoic narratives are often nonsensical. What makes sense is that the body is designed to receive natural, untampered nutrition, including minerals, vitamins, and clean, hydrating water.

The term has evolved into a pursuit of financial gain, where monetary value holds paramount importance and is characterised by an insatiable desire for wealth. In the context of medicine, the term "medication" refers to a substance that exerts a psychological influence on the body. When examining the medical definition of "to medicate," it is described as the act of providing medical treatment or introducing a medical substance into the body. Synonyms for "medicate" include terms such as administer, relax, poison, and treat.

The chemicals used in pharmaceuticals encompass a range of substances, including acetone, diethyl ether, acetic anhydride, toluene, hydrochloric acid, benzyl chloride, along with various other organic compounds.

The seven deadly Sins

The Origins of the Seven Deadly Sins

Betty Little (2023)

In the fourth century, a Christian monk named Evagrius Ponticus documented what are referred to as the "eight evil thoughts": gluttony, lust, avarice, anger, sloth, sadness, vainglory, and pride.

Evagrius' writings were not crafted for a wide readership; instead, as an ascetic monk within the Eastern Christian tradition, his objective was to educate fellow monks on how these eight thoughts could hinder their spiritual pursuits. His disciple, John Cassian, subsequently brought these ideas to the Western Church, where they were translated from Greek into Latin. In the sixth century, St. Gregory the Great, who would later ascend to the papacy as Pope Gregory I, restructured these thoughts in his commentary on the Book of Job, excluding "sloth" and adding "envy."

He also chose not to assign "pride" a separate rank on the list but rather described it as the principal vice that governs the other seven, which ultimately became recognised as the seven deadly sins.

Richard G. Newhauser, an English professor at Arizona State University and editor of works concerning the seven deadly sins, explains, "These sins are referred to as 'mortal' or 'deadly' because they ultimately lead to the demise of the soul. Engaging in any of these mortal sins without seeking confession or performing penance will culminate in the soul's death, resulting in eternal damnation in hell."

In the 13th century, theologian Thomas Aquinas revisited the list of sins in his work *Summa Theologica* ("Summary of Theology"). In his enumeration, he reinstated "sloth" while removing "sadness." Similar to Gregory, Aquinas identified "pride" as the principal sin governing the others. The current capital sins, as outlined in the *Catechism of the Catholic Church*, closely align with Aquinas' list, except that "pride" has supplanted "vainglory."

The seven deadly sins served as a prominent theme in medieval art and literature, which likely contributed to their enduring presence as a concept throughout the ages.

1. **Pride/Vainglory** – Pride is considered the most egregious of the seven deadly sins, often serving as a precursor to other transgressions. This sin is characterised by an individual's belief in their superiority over others, accompanied by excessive admiration for their own accomplishments while failing to recognise the achievements of those around them.

2. **Greed/Avarice** – Newhauser states that Gregory the Great articulated that avarice encompasses not only a longing for material wealth but also for prestige and elevated status. This suggests that what we might deem immaterial can also become the target of avarice. Although the enumeration of sins may differ across various lists, avarice or greed consistently appears in all of them.

3. **Envy** – Clarke notes that while Evagrius does not include envy among his vices, he does address sadness. "Sadness is intricately linked to envy, as envy involves two primary aspects: the pleasure derived from another's misfortune and the grief felt over someone else's success."

4. **Wrath** – Anger may be a natural response to perceived injustice; however, wrath transcends this. The *Catechism* explains that "when anger escalates to a conscious desire to kill or severely harm a neighbour/other, it constitutes a serious violation of charity and is considered a mortal sin." Medieval artists often illustrated wrath through depictions of conflict and instances of suicide.

5. **Lust** – Lust is a concept that extends beyond the confines of heterosexual marriage, encompassing both extramarital and marital sexual relations. The *Catechism* characterises lust as a "disordered desire for or excessive enjoyment of sexual pleasure." Such pleasure is deemed morally disordered when pursued solely for its own sake, detached from its procreative and unitive functions. In contemporary discourse, lust is often perceived as an excessive craving, not only for sexual gratification but also for wealth, fame, or indulgence in food.

6. **Gluttony** – Gluttony refers to the excessive consumption of any substance intended for ingestion or the overindulgence in various items to the extent that it leads to wastefulness.

7. **Sloth** – Sloth is commonly understood as "laziness" in contemporary discourse; however, early Christian theologians interpreted it as "a lack of care in fulfilling spiritual obligations," according to Newhauser. Although Gregory did not explicitly list sloth among the seven deadly sins, he referenced it in the context of sadness or melancholy, noting that such melancholy leads to "slothfulness in fulfilling the commands."

When Aquinas revised the list of capital sins, substituting sloth for sadness, he preserved a link between the two concepts. He articulated that "sloth is a form of sadness," which causes an individual to become lethargic in spiritual practices due to the physical fatigue they induce.

I interpret this from the prayer "Deliver me from evil" as "Deliver me from ego." When we wake up and recognise this, we return to the Garden of Eden, where none of the stories exist. It is a quiet place, an energy that vibrates with peace and love. The recognition that the ego is a phenomenon—it is not real.

What is mental illness. Overall, you can see this in the levels of consciousness has David Hawkins describes.

Self-Identification	Dimension and Colour	Vibration & level of consciousness		
Absolute Self 1000. Supra Causal self-850. Causal Self -800. Universal Self - 700. Galactic Self - 600. Planetary Self - 540. Higher self -539/ 400.	12ᵗʰ Dimension	1000 – full consciousness		
		900 – Supra Causal Truth		
		850 – Devine Grace & Love union		
	Enlightenment	800 – The Gear Void		
		700 – Awareness		
	I AM Presence	670 – Non-Duality		
		600 – Presence		
	5ᵗʰ Dimension	540 – Oneness	Self-Realisation	
	Heaven			
	New humanity consciousness	500 – inner love		
		440 – Inner Wisdom		
		400 – Inner Light		
	Paradise			
Rational linear Emotional Self	4ᵗʰ Dimension	350- Acceptance	Self – Empowerment	
		310 – Willingness		
		250 – Neutrality		
		200 – Courage		
	In-between			
Lower Ego-Self 20 -199	3ʳᵈ Dimension	175 – Pride		
		150 – Anger	Victim/Abuser	
		125 – Desire		
		100 – Fear		
	Purgatory			
	Hell	75 – Grief		
		50 – Apathy		
		30 – Guilt		
		20 – Shame		

Animals.

Animals have often been perceived as dangerous, which may reflect our own fears and projections. In contrast, their prey thrives in the wild, enjoying a life of freedom and happiness. Conversely, our prey is subjected to confinement, mistreatment, medication, and stress, ultimately leading to their slaughter for our consumption.

We ingest not only the flesh but also the trauma, stress hormones, and substances administered to these animals. Idoni posits that cannibalism should be avoided, which we interpret as refraining from consuming one another.

However, if we were intended to consume living beings, why do we not hunt them with our teeth and eat them raw, as animals do? Furthermore, why do we label them, instead of acknowledging the truth—that we are eating a dead, mutated body pumped with chemicals to reduce rotting?

According to the *Gospel of the Holy Twelve*, it is stated that Jesus did not consume any living beings. He admonished those who partake in the consumption of the flesh and blood of any creature of the sky, land, or sea, or those who drink strong beverages. He also warned against harming the creatures entrusted to humanity by God. He urged individuals to refrain from hunting innocent beings and to purify themselves from wicked actions, for those who do so are unworthy of receiving the higher mysteries.

Wild animals exist in a state of freedom, savouring the natural provisions available to them until they meet their end, whether through natural causes or predation. For centuries, narratives have been woven around animals. Have we not observed that animals inhabited this planet long before us, that nature thrived independently of human influence, and that these creatures once lived in a harmonious paradise?

I have come to understand that animals embody love and forgiveness, yet we impose collars around their necks and adorn them in frivolous attire to conform to our societal norms. In the wild, I have never encountered an animal's hair, fur, or feathers turning grey with wrinkles or showing signs of ageing or deterioration.

Although monkeys and chimpanzees develop grey hair, their greying stops at a certain age and is not necessarily an indication of ageing. Have you ever seen a bird going grey? Instead, I see the animal's maturity. They are genuine, robust, and possess an appropriate physique.

Animals do not require vaccinations, medications, or chemicals. It appears that only domesticated animals—confined, subjected to processed foods, and kept for our amusement—face such interventions. They endure our presence, and when they resist, we resort to lethal measures. Unlike humans, they do not subscribe to a fabricated narrative of intelligence; they embody intelligence itself, fully aware and awake, unencumbered by the delusions of a restless ego imposed by their captors.

Isabell Thomas

My Poems.

The Ego

I lay there in this wonderful place

Around me, there is no time, just space

My body lets go of the world that I am in

I let go of my ego, that troublesome thing.

The ego is not stable; it says what's not true,

And it keeps me from peace, from the wonderful you.

I can leave the ego at any time,

But I was taught to believe that the ego is mine.

It is just a recording that is in my brain,

Which plays the same negatives over again.

Its drives me nuts and sometimes crazy

But the stories sound as fresh as a daisy.

I listen to them as if they are new,

But the stories are a repeat and not always true.

If I asked the ego, who are you talking to?

It never answers, "I am talking to you."

That is when I recognise the divide,

And a split from the ego goes on inside.

Our egos are not stable; it creates a story, a saying, and a label.

Like the 'not been good enough' that is not true,

But if I don't have a good enough story,

How can I give one to you?

We hear ego stories and we hold them inside,

Sometimes with dislike them, or hold them with pride,

People say, what's been said to them, and we repeat these stories over again.

My ego feeds off of my interest. I give notoriety to this pest.

The world is made up of an ego state; it tells us a story,

It predicts our fate.

But can this story be really true?

When the ego is not you?

When I let it go and remove the vail. I observe its lies and never-ending tale.

The feelings that come along are the ego too, that's what makes the stories feel true.

If we eat unhealthy food it shapes, our health, our body and mood.

That is the same for the psychological food.

How much did you feed yourself today, and give your egoic brain to play?

How many other egos do you listen to?

That change your mood and shape you?

Reconcile and release, don't blame the ego, send it peace.

The ego thoughts are like clouds in the sky, they often change and pass you bye. Another cloud may come and look the same, let it pass when it comes again.

I listened to the world outside of me that told me what I am and who I should be. That creates anxiety.

Maybe it's not true,

Instead

I was born to do me and not to do you,

To do what others said I should do.

Maybe that is an egoic story that you told to me,

Because that egoic story was told to you?

Isabell Thomas 2024

Bullying

When I first laid my eyes on you, I believed everything you taught me was true.

My brain was set and ready to go, with all of the knowledge that you could show.

I lived my life with anger inside. With hate and lies and full of pride.

I could not find a space to grow, my space was filled with what 'you' know.

I communicated with what you taught me, a fist a shout, with misery.

My interactions with others were key, to match the same way you had with me.

My skin was grey, my hands were sore, my body ached, I could punch no more.

People looked at me with fear in their eyes, I knew their smiles were a disguise.

I hated me and they did too. I guess in the same way that, I hated you.

I took pleasure in seeing the pain in others, then I could hide my pain under my covers.

I could hear my voice, it sounded like you, when I ordered my victims what to do.

I remember when you did that to me, in my younger years of misery.

I found love sometimes though fleeting and passed, as my anger would come out from behind the mask.

I just wanted love, but who would love me, it was something I could never see.

I thought the world was the problem, and that the world hated me, so I went to sort out the world by going to therapy.

Through therapy, I had begun to see. I was using the gifts you had given me.

I learnt those gifts were not all you, you had been given the same gifts too.

I have learnt not to do what you did to me. I learn to take responsibility.

What is inside of me is what I give out. I heard your insides; they would always shout.

This is not how I was meant to be. They were the unwanted gifts you gave to me.

I have emptied my insides of most of you, and I take accountability for what I do.

I hold my hands up and set myself free.

I will no longer be the Man, you taught me to be.

Isabell Thomas 2023

Deliver me from Evil.

We have attempted to transform ourselves into entities that create divisions among us, competing with one another by dehumanising ourselves in order to feel unique through various ideologies. Those who perceive themselves as superior have exposed their patterns of abuse, seeking to inflate their evil/egos, as their self-worth is contingent upon drawing validation from others, much like a parasite.

The so-called superior individuals are merely human beings engaging in abusive behaviours. They have manifested their own afflictions but project these issues onto others to avoid confronting their true selves.

Our uniqueness lies in the fact that we are devoid of labels, names, or the ego. As Shakespeare noted, *"The world is a stage, and we are all acting on it."* We are remarkable because we share a fundamental connection with everything in the universe. When did we cease to be a part of nature?

It is essential to discover who you are beyond your actions or the perceptions others hold of you. How can others truly understand your essence if they lack self-awareness? They often merely echo words that have been imparted to them, leaving one to question their authenticity.

Some may notice your departure from a particular role. For instance, if you engage in substance abuse, you are responding to an experience, mistakenly identifying yourself with that experience and thus embodying it. You resort to substance use to prolong that experience, further developing your role as either a victim or perpetrator, or sometimes both.

You align yourself with others in a similar, homogeneous group, collectively enacting your roles. This dynamic can be distressing, occasionally providing fleeting pleasure, yet the ego remains unstable, ever-changing, and perpetually desiring. It acts as a master, demanding your attention; without your engagement, it cannot endure, as it lacks true existence.

Choosing to cease substance use signifies a refusal to continue nourishing that aspect of your ego. Consequently, you must detach from the homogeneous group, for leaving that part of your ego necessitates distancing yourself from theirs as well.

We still follow those who have professional labels, but I must reiterate that a professional label does not eliminate or override human egoic thinking. This is evident in some of the appalling behaviours you may have heard of or experienced.

I have encountered professionals who refuse to think beyond their own doctrines, opting to overlook alternative approaches. This signifies a lack of awareness regarding the exploration of new possibilities or a refusal to engage with them—particularly when such alternatives may not have proven advantageous for those who benefit from programming individuals.

As previously articulated in this text, our actions are often dictated by external instructions or societal expectations, which constrain our autonomy both in our internal psyche and in the external environment governed by the egos of others. True freedom resides within.

We cannot unlearn what has been learned, yet one can choose to remain wilfully bound to that knowledge. However, the act of seeing cannot be undone. It has become clear to me that the processes of buying and selling require a story, particularly when we ourselves are the focal point. The absence of humanity would render buying and selling non-existent. We can change these acts when we change our beliefs.

Rather than seeking guidance from the creator of this planet, we often turn our attention to the human ego. This ego tends to attribute blame to external factors, embodying a narcissistic perspective, while it is, in reality, accountable for the harm it inflicts. This state of consciousness, as described by David Hawkins, represents a lower vibrational level often referred to as *Hell*. This vibration permeates humanity, influenced by ego-driven programming from television, social media, and news outlets.

We absorb this negativity, allowing it to affect us, and subsequently, we propagate it. I frequently express to those around me that I refrain from consuming news, as it predominantly consists of negative reports, yet they often feel compelled to share such news with me. We collectively inhabit this *Hell*, transmitting its essence from one individual to another, and we inadvertently teach our children this mindset through our actions and words.

The ego tends to blame nature in order to promote products, neglecting to scrutinise the products and chemicals themselves. How misguided is the ego to assert that nature is detrimental while deeming artificial products and chemicals beneficial?

Humans lack the capability to create a plant; we can only speculate about its formation. How can a species that considers itself intelligent accept this notion while remaining followers?

We tend to follow the news and accept much of what is presented without verifying its accuracy. Envision individuals on social media mimicking each other in real life—one might feel stalked, harassed, or simply realise that they are all aimlessly circling one another. If one were to observe people walking in a circle, following each other without purpose, as they do on social media, what conclusions might one draw from such behaviour?

It is important to recognise that we do not possess the ability to create the universe, plant life, nature, or living beings, including humans. However, the inflated sense of ego among humans has led to the invention of labels, narratives, and a misguided sense of superiority and control.

One of the most significant narratives is the tendency to blame the creator of the universe. This perspective criticises the essence of life itself, suggesting a false superiority over it.

For instance, the claim that one can heal ailments caused by the sun through chemicals or surgical procedures is misleading. The assertion that one can rejuvenate skin or provide essential nutrients is often based on belief rather than truth.

Furthermore, the notion that artificially enhanced food is superior to what nature provides is flawed, as it often involves the use of harmful substances such as pesticides and genetically modified organisms.

When individuals experience health issues or weight gain, the blame is frequently placed on them for consuming the very foods that have been marketed to them. These foods may not adequately nourish the body, leading to persistent hunger signals, compounded by the addition of sugar that fosters addiction. The body, in its effort to survive, may redistribute food away from vital organs, resulting in increased body size.

Moreover, individuals are often inundated with chemicals through personal care products and household cleaners, many of which are marketed under well-known brands. These products, despite their claims of containing vitamins, are often synthetic and can be harmful. In contrast, natural alternatives, such as organic fruit juices, offer a more beneficial option without the presence of chemicals.

The deterioration of health is frequently misattributed to ageing when, in reality, it is often a consequence of a diet filled with human-made chemicals rather than natural foods. Society tends to focus on what is perceived as wrong with individuals rather than promoting what is beneficial for their health and the environment. Those who prioritise profit over the well-being of the planet and its inhabitants contribute to this misguided narrative.

Changing What You Have Been Programmed With.

Humanity has cultivated—or been born into—a belief system that undermines both the human and animal kingdoms, reducing us all to mere commodities for profit. We find ourselves divided by species, race, colour—whether of skin or hair—weight, social class, appearance, sexuality, and age.

Your mind is your own, even if you may not fully realise it. I recall a university lecturer who used the story of an elephant tethered by a rope as a metaphor for the human condition. The lecturer recounted how a young elephant was captured and confined, exploited for profit in a circus.

The elephant was rewarded with food for compliance and punished through beatings or starvation for disobedience. Over time, the elephant learned to submit to the man's demands. Despite its physical growth, the elephant failed to recognise that it was not only larger than the man but also stronger than the rope that bound it.

The elephant could have easily overpowered the man and broken free from its restraints. Instead, it constructed a mental prison—one that mirrored its physical confinement—having forgotten its true identity and accepted the role of both prisoner and servant.

The lecturer's message was clear: we, as human beings, are similarly entrapped. We too have created a prison within a prison. The mental confines we experience stem from:

1. What we have learned about our surroundings, and

2. Our external experiences.

Our perceptions of the world are shaped by both factors. In this process, we have not only lost sight of who we are but seldom take the time to inquire about it.

The Wooden Table.

I often share with my clients the story of the wooden table.

When observing a wooden table, one may notice its shape and size, as well as the various objects placed upon it. Is this table a source of pride for you, or has it become a repository for unwanted items? Has it been painted over due to a dislike for its original colour, or do you appreciate the visibility of its natural grain through a layer of varnish?

Upon closer inspection, can you see reflections of yourself in the table? Consider how you have been influenced, the burdens you carry, and the treatment you have received. Do others seek to alter your essence or vitality, or do they wish to appreciate you as you are, through their own lens?

Similar to the table, you were not created in your current form. Just as the table originated from a tree, you are not merely a product of societal expectations; you are a spirit. You have been distanced from your true self. As the table is no longer identified as a tree— its source—so too is the human no longer recognised as a spirit or a human being, our source. Instead, we have been shaped by labels and have become "human-doings"—actors or actresses, as Shakespeare noted—performing roles assigned by our labels.

Those confined within a prison can only impart their understanding of that environment, including its rules and expectations. When we begin to undervalue ourselves, we inadvertently teach others the same lessons we have learned. But for whom are you conforming if it means straying from your authentic self?

We often find ourselves preoccupied with fulfilling the roles dictated by others, who may not have our best interests at heart. This behaviour extends to how we treat our homes, plants, and the life around us.

The Sabbath

The Sabbath represents the sacred day of rest that our Creator established upon completing His work of creation. This leads me to contemplate the concept of "human-doing" and the purpose behind our actions. God has accomplished everything for our benefit, allowing us to relish our experiences on this Earth.

There is no need for us to seek or labour for happiness; it is inherently ours. Similarly, we do not need to study to attain intelligence, as it is already within us. Our brains function as recording devices, capturing information for later recall; this process should not be mistaken for intelligence, which is merely the act of remembering. We receive recognition for recalling knowledge that God has already provided.

Those who are mentally unwell may not recognise their condition, as they have come to accept it as normal, as noted by Freud (1855) and Fromm (1944).

Delusion?

I frequently encounter individuals proclaiming, "Let us make Britain great again." This prompts me to question: when exactly was Britain great, and for whom was it deemed so?

From my experience and observations, some are born into a constrained existence, subservient to those who confine us. However, upon gaining awareness of this reality, we cease to be mere victims of our circumstances and instead become active participants, ultimately victimising ourselves.

This is often due to the collar around our necks, which contains words like *must*, *should*, *have to*, *got to*, and *fear*. It is a disservice to humanity for one individual to expect another to follow them, especially when it is not they who provide for our needs. Our true sustenance comes from our Creator, who supplies all that we are and all that we require. Yet, we often choose to follow those who have constructed labels and categorised the world around us, weaving narratives filled with falsehoods.

Time and again, we turn to the same individuals, only to receive the same outcomes repeatedly, failing to recognise a way to break free from this cycle. We have placed our trust in these figures, leading us deeper into a metaphorical rabbit hole, often at the expense of our well-being.

We rely on the FDA to oversee the safety of our food supply, and while they do regulate it, we have grown accustomed to consuming substances labelled as food, which are, in fact, laden with chemicals. When these chemicals adversely affect our health, we resort to more chemicals in the form of medication to numb the signals our bodies send us regarding the harm being inflicted upon it. We willingly choose ignorance, valuing professional labels or flavours that we have been conditioned to accept as pleasurable.

Belief in God, our Creator, transcends religion; it embodies a way of life characterised by unity with oneself and nature, fostering harmony. When one achieves inner harmony, they resonate with the broader universe. Conversely, if one is in conflict with themselves, they will find themselves at odds with everything around them.

The world we inhabit reflects our actions and the roles we assume based on our beliefs. These roles are not dictated by our experiences or the opinions of others; rather, they are merely the transmission of knowledge—whether positive, negative, or neutral—that others have imparted to us.

It is important to emphasise that we have strayed significantly from our true essence, transforming into individuals who merely fulfil the desires of those around us. These individuals often act out of self-interest, driven by want, greed, conflict, control, and abuse.

They adopt various titles and engage in actions that perpetuate evil. For instance, those who provide us with food may conspire to compromise its quality, ultimately harming our health for profit.

Similarly, while some individuals in the medical field genuinely seek to heal, others may prioritise financial gain, aligning themselves with the pharmaceutical industry.

Furthermore, certain law enforcement officers may actively seek out conflict, contributing to its creation and supporting those who desire control. There are also individuals who enact laws that contradict the principles established by our Creator, motivated by financial incentives.

Shahid Bolsen (2024) speaks about how:

"So-called Western civilisation is a myth, and you are not going to find any solutions as long as you hold on to any belief in that fiction. Your history does not contain any guidance for you except in so far as it shows you, very clearly, how not to be. You need to stop digging in those empty pockets. If you dig into the pockets of Western history, all you're going to do is get your hands stained with blood."

Our ancestors adopted the perspective that violence and dominance were the sole means of survival. Bolsen illustrated how elements of primitive society can be observed at various levels within Western culture. It was believed that taking from others equated to merit, reflecting a culture that prioritises outcomes over methods.

In an attempt to conceal the truth, the West feigned civility when encountering authentic civilisations, pretending to uphold values and principles that they neither genuinely adhere to nor comprehend. This has led to a state of cognitive dissonance, stemming from the unblemished human nature inherent in all individuals.

Satan Tempts Jesus

"4 Then Jesus was led up by the Spirit into the wilderness to be tempted by the devil.

2 And when He had fasted forty days and forty nights, afterward He was hungry.

3 Now when the tempter came to Him, he said, "If You are the Son of God, command that these stones become bread."

4 But He answered and said, "It is written, 'Man shall not live by bread alone, but by every word that proceeds from the mouth of God.'

5 Then the devil took Him up into the holy city, set Him on the pinnacle of the temple,

6 and said to Him, "If You are the Son of God, throw Yourself down. For it is written:

'He shall give His angels charge over you,'

and, 'In their hands they shall bear you up,

Lest you dash your foot against a stone.'"

7 Jesus said to him, "It is written again, 'You shall not [a]tempt the Lord your God.'"

8 Again, the devil took Him up on an exceedingly high mountain, and showed Him all the kingdoms of the world and their glory.

⁹ *And he said to Him, "All these things I will give You if You will fall down and worship me."*

¹⁰ *Then Jesus said to him,* [b] *"Away with you, Satan! For it is written, 'You shall worship the Lord your God, and Him only you shall serve.'"*

¹¹ *Then the devil left Him, and behold, angels came and ministered to Him."*

Satan in Mankind

It is a profound manipulation to convince humanity to desire all the resources of the planet for individual gain, leading to the destruction of the creations of our originators. This includes acts of cannibalism, killing, imprisonment, torture, and experimentation on these beings.

We shift the blame onto the Sun for our ailments, attributing our discontent to nature and our own physical forms, perpetually seeking satisfaction that eludes us. If one were to embody the role of an evil force, would they not incite humanity to engage in such madness, exploiting them to obliterate the very creations of our Creator, of which we are all a part? We have become both conscious and unconscious participants in the harm we inflict upon others and ourselves.

The abuse of oneself inevitably translates into the abuse of others—whether it be oneself, one's children, fellow humans, or creatures—as our actions resonate within us and are perceived by others, manifesting in various levels of awareness.

We have been conditioned to exhibit traits akin to Stockholm syndrome, wherein we develop trust in our captors, accept their harmful offerings as delightful treats, and seek assistance from those who inflict pain upon us, labelling some of their toxic substances as medicine. Our participation in these dynamics stems from a reluctance to assume responsibility for our own lives. This is apparent when people often ask:

- *What should I do?*
- *How will life be?*
- *What should I eat instead?*

These questions reveal an absence of self-sovereignty and autonomy. Furthermore, the phenomenon of *change blindness* significantly contributes to our failure to recognise or acknowledge the ongoing changes in our circumstances and environment. This occurs due to the misplaced trust we place in others and our tendency to disempower ourselves.

Change blindness, a concept in psychology, refers to the inability to notice alterations in one's surroundings, often resulting from a lack of attention. This unawareness can manifest when changes are subtle or unexpected, or when individuals are focused on other tasks.

For example, one might miss significant changes in a rapidly alternating image or fail to notice a person's change in attire due to distractions elsewhere in the scene. This phenomenon is prevalent as we consume information from news outlets and social media, which continually divert our attention from the underlying truths and direct us in ways that serve those who wish to manipulate our beliefs and thoughts.

Among the many gifts bestowed upon us at birth, two of the most significant are **vibration** and **imagination**. Our vibration and imagination shape our reality, as the entire world is a product of imagination. Nothing in existence was created without first being envisioned.

However, we are often taught from a young age that using our imagination is inappropriate. For instance, have you ever been told that you or your child is a daydreamer and should cease such behaviour? Instead, we tend to conform to the daydreams imposed by others, which often reflect a narrative of control and subservience to a master.

Is There Something More at Work?

Looking at biblical texts reveals that God has killed over 300 million people in the Bible, while Satan is not recorded as having killed anybody. The Bible also reveals that there is more than one God.

The *King James Bible*, Genesis (John 1:1-5), states:

"God said, let us make man in our image."

Who was that God talking to?

Genesis 1:28 further states:

"And God blessed them, and God said unto them, be fruitful, and multiply, and replenish the earth, and subdue it: and have dominion over the fish of the sea, and over the fowl of the air, and over every living thing that moveth upon the earth."

This does not speak about the Creator of all. I understand this to be a god speaking to a god.

We have been **subdued**, meaning: *depressed, muted, low in spirit, dejected*. Not only that, but:

"The devil took Him up on an exceedingly high mountain, and showed Him all the kingdoms of the world and their glory. And he said to Him, 'All these things I will give You if You will fall down and worship me.'"

This reveals that the ego's wants are tied to the things of the earth—things we have made valuable through fabricated stories that fuel our never-ending thirst, keeping us trapped in the *hell consciousness*.

Our History.

Throughout the world, one can observe various power centres and institutions of learning. These locations often bear the marks of deliberate destruction. The Anunnaki, a pantheon of deities revered by the ancient Sumerians, Akkadians, Assyrians, and Babylonians, are central to this narrative. It is believed that humanity existed prior to the arrival of the Anunnaki, who were regarded as divine beings. In biblical texts, it is stated: *"Let us make man in our image,"* indicating the relationship between humans and these gods.

In exchange for offerings, humanity sought knowledge from deities such as Enki, the god associated with creation, knowledge, and craftsmanship, as well as Thoth, the Egyptian god of wisdom, writing, and magic. The insights imparted to humanity, particularly regarding the cosmos, were believed to originate from these divine entities.

It is useful to know why the work of Zecharia Sitchin is so important, as it is from his ideas that the Kings of England derived the concept of a *divine right*. Zecharia Sitchin (July 11, 1920 – October 9, 2010) was a prolific author known for his works exploring human origins through the lens of ancient astronaut theories.

He posited that the Anunnaki, a race of extraterrestrial beings from a distant planet named Nibiru, were responsible for the emergence of the ancient Sumerian civilisation. According to Sitchin, Sumerian mythology indicates that Nibiru follows an elongated elliptical orbit around the Sun, taking approximately 3,600 years to complete a single revolution.

According to Sitchin, Enki, the Sumerian deity associated with water and human civilisation, proposed the creation of primitive workers (Homo sapiens) through genetic engineering. He asserts that the beings referred to as the Nephilim in the *Book of Genesis* emerged following the entry of Nibiru into the inner Solar System.

He theorises that they arrived on Earth approximately 450,000 years ago in search of minerals, particularly gold, which they discovered and extracted in Africa. Sitchin proposed that these "gods" were the ordinary labourers involved in the colonial mission to Earth from the planet Nibiru. This initiative aimed to alleviate the burden on the Anunnaki, who had revolted due to their dissatisfaction with working conditions, by producing slaves to replace them in the gold mines. This was to be achieved by combining extraterrestrial genes with those of *Homo erectus*.

Sitchin asserts that ancient inscriptions indicate human civilisation in Sumer, Mesopotamia, was established under the oversight of these "gods," with the institution of human kingship serving as a means to connect humanity with the Anunnaki, thereby giving rise to the doctrine of the *divine right of kings*.

Furthermore, Sitchin posits that the destructive *"evil wind"* mentioned in the *Lament for Ur*, which led to the downfall of Ur around 2000 BCE, was a consequence of nuclear fallout from a conflict among extraterrestrial groups, with the precise date of this event being 2024 BCE. He contends that his findings align with numerous biblical texts, which he claims are derived from earlier Sumerian writings.

Akhenaten and the Shift to Monotheism

Ancient Egypt flourished during the 14th century BCE, with religion playing a significant role in the lives of the Egyptians. A pharaoh named Akhenaten, originally named Amenhotep (meaning *"Amun is content"*), was the second son of Amenhotep III and his principal wife, Queen Tiye.

Following the unexpected death of his older brother, Thutmose, in his youth, Amenhotep ascended to the throne. After the death of his father in 1353 BCE, Amenhotep was crowned pharaoh as Amenhotep IV in Thebes, becoming the tenth ruler of the 18th dynasty. He married the renowned Nefertiti, who became his *Great Royal Wife*.

Despite having multiple wives, records indicate that Nefertiti and Amenhotep shared a close and intimate bond, resulting in six daughters but no sons. Nefertiti emerged as a highly influential queen, enjoying her position as the second most powerful individual in Egypt.

Akhenaten sought to overturn centuries of tradition by compelling the Egyptian populace to abandon their polytheistic beliefs in favour of the worship of a single deity, Aten. Although he was branded a rebel and a heretic, he introduced the revolutionary concept of monotheism (the doctrine that there is one God), which significantly altered the course of history.

Amun was the central deity of numerous cults during this period, which, despite their diverse gods and practices, generally emphasised balance and eternal harmony. The cult of Amun had been gaining strength and influence for centuries, and by the time of the new pharaoh's reign, they had amassed considerable wealth and status, rivalling that of the royal family. In fact, it is said that the priests of Amun owned more land than the pharaoh himself. This situation may have contributed to Akhenaten's desire to challenge the established order.

For the first five years of his reign, he permitted the worship of all traditional Egyptian gods. However, likely influenced by his mother, Queen Tiye, the pharaoh's focus gradually shifted toward one particular deity—Aten.

Aten is primarily characterised as the solar disc, originally associated with the sun god Ra. It is artistically represented as a disc emitting rays, each ending in small hands. The renowned *Stele of Akhenaten* illustrates the royal family receiving the rays of Aten. While the worship of Aten was not unparalleled—previously, Pharaoh Amenhotep III had honoured Aten above all other deities— his son Akhenaten took this devotion to an unprecedented level.

To signify his commitment to Aten, he changed his name in the fifth year of his reign from Amenhotep IV to Akhenaten, meaning *"living spirit of Aten."* By the ninth year of his rule, Akhenaten proclaimed Aten not only as the supreme deity but as the sole object of worship.

This radical declaration is often regarded as a precursor to monotheism; however, Atenism is more accurately described as *monolatry* or *henotheism*, as its adherents acknowledged the existence of other lesser gods while focusing their worship on a single deity.

Akhenaten ordered the defacement and destruction of temples dedicated to Amun and prohibited the representation of any god other than Aten. He had references to other deities removed from monuments throughout Egypt.

Furthermore, Akhenaten asserted that he was the sole messenger of Aten, effectively displacing priests and other religious authorities. The aristocracy perceived this abrupt shift towards monotheism as a considerable threat to the empire, yet they largely complied with the Pharaoh's modifications.

Some priests of Amun managed to preserve texts and artefacts, shielding them from Akhenaten's wrath. Towards the end of his reign, Akhenaten went so far as to declare himself and Nefertiti as actual deities, demanding worship in their names. Meanwhile, the populace labelled the Pharaoh a heretic king and regarded him as a puritanical tyrant who had abolished Egypt's religious freedoms.

The Pharaoh commanded the establishment of a new capital, which he named Akhetaten, signifying "Horizon of Aten." This city, commonly referred to as Amarna in its Arabic designation, was strategically located in the heart of Egypt, positioned between the ancient centres of power in Thebes and Memphis. Akhenaten envisioned Amarna as a remote site where he could cultivate a new religion, free from the persistent influences of the traditional deities.

He constructed monuments and temples without roofs, permitting sunlight to illuminate the worshippers directly.

The Pharaoh's name is still referenced today. At the end of a prayer, when you say 'Amen', you are invoking Akhenaten.

King James Bible, Exodus 20:5:

"Thou shalt not bow down thyself to them, nor serve them: for I, the LORD thy God, am a jealous God, visiting the iniquity of the fathers upon the children unto the third and fourth generation of them that hate me."

Meaning: Visiting the evil of the fathers upon the children.

What Measures Does Satan Employ Against the Light Embodied by Jesus?

He faces ridicule, contempt, ostracism, slander, and mockery. The truth is frequently met with resistance. Jesus proclaims himself as the Son of God, drawing a comparison to the sun, which illuminates the world and cannot be possessed by any individual. The sun represents our risen saviour, as it fosters the abundance of life for all.

In 1993, Philip Donahue engaged in a discussion regarding the debate over Jesus's racial identity, with Blair Underwood portraying Jesus. Underwood noted that throughout Jesus's lineage, all individuals were people of colour.

He also emphasised that colour is fundamentally "a matter of the heart," suggesting that at our core, we share the same essence. The divisions among us arise from our narratives.

Ultimately, depicting Jesus as white serves to reinforce white supremacy, a theme that has persisted throughout history. The injustices faced by Jesus parallel the destruction of statues in Egypt that depicted gods of colour—a process initiated by Akhenaten and repeated throughout history. This pattern continued during slavery, including the erasure of contributions made by Black inventors.

To claim supremacy does not equate to possessing power over others; rather, it signifies deceit, violence, and betrayal, as one is armed with the tools to enact such roles, which Satan tempts individuals to embrace.

Theologians and cultural institutions have suppressed the belief that Jesus was Black. Most people believe that Jesus was Caucasian with light hair and blue eyes. However, this image does not align with the region where he lived.

Jesus's connections to history, the Bible, and Africa are significant. He was born in Bethlehem, located in Roman-occupied Judea. As a Middle Eastern Jew, Jesus's heritage links him to a region that serves as a crossroads for three continents: Africa, Asia, and Europe. In ancient times, this area was characterised by a rich diversity.

The Gospel of Matthew highlights the clear ties to Africa, noting that Joseph received a divine warning in a dream, prompting him to take Mary and the infant Jesus to Egypt for their safety, thereby fleeing King Herod's lethal decree.

Egypt, a North African nation, provided refuge for the Jewish people, particularly during periods of persecution, such as the Babylonian exile. This historical context underscores the profound connection between Jesus and his family and the African continent. Egypt was inhabited by individuals of African descent, suggesting that Mary, Joseph, and Jesus would have blended into this society due to shared physical characteristics.

Had they been Caucasian, they likely would have attracted undue attention. Ancient representations of Jesus from Egypt and Ethiopia depict him with dark skin, textured hair, and distinctly African features, supporting the notion of his African ancestry.

This belief has influenced Ethiopian culture for centuries. The Gospels also mention Simon of Cyrene, who assisted Jesus in carrying his cross, identifying him as a North African figure. This challenges the prevalent Western portrayal of a white Jesus, which has historically reinforced colonial ambitions and white supremacy.

The depiction of Jesus as a Caucasian figure emerged around the 15th century. In 2024, Russian President Vladimir Putin announced the unveiling of a secret vault containing paintings of Jesus, the Virgin Mary, King Solomon, and Elisha, all portrayed as Black. However, there is debate as to whether this is true.

Additionally, his family and those surrounding him, including angels, were also depicted as Black. Putin has commissioned sacred icons from a museum to be displayed in a Moscow cathedral. This collection, known as the Russian Icons, comprises hundreds of paintings that narrate the life of Jesus and the historical context of that era.

In the early centuries of Christianity, aniconism—the rejection of religious images—significantly influenced Christian art. However, this perspective was eventually abandoned during the Byzantine period, leading to diverse representations of Jesus. One of the earliest depictions was that of the Good Shepherd, which evolved into the portrayal of Jesus as a figure with blonde hair and blue eyes.

It does not seem fitting to describe Jesus as looking Caucasian, as this may have been used to justify the enslavement of Africans.

Christianity is often perceived as a means for individuals to assert their moral superiority. However, it raises the question of how this perspective can be held by those who have committed wrongful acts or who adhere to the doctrines outlined in the scripture itself.

Many religions, including Christianity, can be seen as instruments of control, which diverges from the true teachings of Jesus Christ. For instance, in Africa, Christianity has been an integral part of life and predates European influence. The Ethiopian Bible predates the King James Bible.

When missionaries arrived in southern Africa, the acceptance of Christianity by Africans was largely due to the alignment of certain values between Western religion and their own beliefs. Subsequently, the French and British colonisers arrived.

In northern Nigeria and Egypt, Islam is predominantly practised, largely due to the coercive measures employed to convert the local populations. The choice presented to them was stark: accept the faith or face death, as a Muslim army was engaged in what they termed a Holy War or Jihad.

The Ethiopians believe that the relationship between Jesus and the individual is deeply personal, emphasising that Christ resides within each person rather than solely within the pages of a book preached by others. This connection is depicted through a genuine unity of love between each individual and Jesus, which is a tangible spiritual experience.

Nevertheless, the teachings of Christianity have often emerged from a spiritually impoverished context in the West. The only consensus appears to be that certain values are aligned.

Neil deGrasse Tyson (2018) asserts that if a deity exists, then this entity is neither entirely benevolent nor omnipotent, as evidenced by the suffering experienced by humanity. This perspective underlines the concept of faith in religion, which entails believing in something without empirical evidence. Tyson further elaborates, stating, *"As the area of our knowledge expands, so too does the boundary of our ignorance"* (2023).

Additionally, Richard Dawkins (2024) suggests that instead of relying on childhood fantasies, one should examine their own beliefs regarding the world, life, and the universe. Are these beliefs founded on rational justification, or are they merely a product of one's upbringing?

For instance, consider a scenario where three young children portray the three wise men: Shadbreet, a Sikh; Musharraf, a Muslim; and Adele, a Christian. If Shadbreet were depicted as a Monetarist, Musharraf as a Keynesian, and Adele as a Marxist, would it not raise concerns about their parents' suitability to raise children? Does it challenge ethical standards to impose a parent's views onto their offspring?

There are many gods of worship, yet neither the gods nor our worship and behaviour truly reflect love, freedom, truth, equality, respect, or health.

King James Version - Genesis 1:26-28

"26 And God said, Let us make man in our image, after our likeness: and let them have dominion over the fish of the sea, and over the fowl of the air, and over the cattle, and over all the earth, and over every creeping thing that creepeth upon the earth.

27 So God created man in his own image, in the image of God created he him; male and female created he them.

28 And God blessed them, and God said unto them, Be fruitful, and multiply, and replenish the earth, and subdue it: and have

255

dominion over the fish of the sea, and over the fowl of the air, and over every living thing that moveth upon the earth."

The teachings of Jesus appear to contradict Genesis 1:26-28, as his message emphasises love for oneself, for one another, and for all living beings. While Jesus was near Tiberias in Israel, a young man approached him, bringing live pigeons and rabbits to share with Jesus and his disciples. Jesus gazed upon the young man with love and remarked:

"You possess a kind heart, and God shall illuminate your path.

However, do you not understand that God, in the beginning, provided man with the fruits of the earth for sustenance?

He did not create man to be inferior to the ox, horse, or sheep, allowing him to kill and consume the flesh and blood of his fellow beings. Indeed, you believe that creatures should be sacrificed and eaten, but the time will come when your sacrifices and blood feasts shall cease... therefore, let these creatures go free."

(The Gospel of the Holy Twelve, 2024)

This suggests that the teachings of Jesus are derived from the Creator—the Father/Mother God—who resides within us. One might question the difference between God and Satan or whose image we are truly made in, considering historical behaviours.

As a spiritual entity, I do not subscribe to any particular religion. I seek the Creator within myself, as we are all designed to be sovereign, autonomous, and self-governing individuals, free from oppression and control.

While humanity cannot create life, we often find ourselves enslaved by human words and the teachings of the Bible. The world appears to be governed by external forces. One must consider: if we were meant to be controlled and harmed, why does the body and spirit resist?

Many choose to evade responsibility, instead placing blame on others.

Our growth stems from an inner consciousness rooted in grace. True development cannot arise from being controlled, instructed, dictated to, ruled, manipulated, lied to, and instilled with fear. The Creator resides within us, and our relationship with this Creator is paramount. It is not defined by the ego-driven internal dialogue shaped by external influences and the dictates of humanity.

Human beings are inherently good; however, we are exposed to evil. Consequently, we embark on a quest for goodness, liberty, and happiness, having been misled. We often ignore the true message that arises within us through our pain, illness, discomfort, and unhappiness. These feelings signal that we are acting against our true nature and consuming—physically, mentally, and emotionally—what we should not.

Upon introspection, we discover our passions, tranquillity, affection, and the essence of our Creator.

Isabell Thomas

What's Happened to Our Human Rights?

Human rights advocates agree that, six decades after its adoption, the Universal Declaration of Human Rights remains largely an aspiration rather than a reality. Violations are prevalent across the globe. For instance, Amnesty International's *2009 World Report* and various other sources indicate that individuals are:

- Subjected to torture or mistreatment in at least 81 nations.

- Enduring unjust trials in at least 54 nations.

- Facing restrictions on their freedom of expression in at least 77 nations.

Moreover, women and children are particularly marginalised in numerous respects, the press is often not free in many regions, and protesters are silenced, frequently with fatal consequences. Although some progress has been achieved over the past sixty years, human rights violations continue to afflict the world today.

.

Conclusion.

Manifestation

There must be an infinite power that runs through all of creation and laws, permeating the entire universe. What is the source behind all of this? What do you call it? Not that it truly matters, as we can all agree that we feel or have an innate knowing that this source is the creator of all.

We are made in the likeness of our creator. What we think, we make true. We are born into a disconnection from our real world. Those who are born into slavery do not know they are slaves. What we have done is create a world governed by a slaver.

The enslaved often ask, *What shall we do if we do not live like this?* We are taught to look up to others. This, in itself, reinforces the idea that we are children, always looking upwards. However, when we turn inward, we encounter the chattering ego, echoing the voices, lies, judgments, and controls of others. When we observe this, we realise it is not our true selves speaking. Looking beyond that, we find peace.

Individuals entrenched in the material realm often engage solely in human action, while those who have attained self-actualisation dwell in the spiritual domain. In the realm of action, the spirit merely observes human endeavours. However, in the spiritual realm, one exists in harmony with nature and possesses self-awareness, recognising the unity of infinite life.

When we surrender to the flow of life and align with its rhythms, we experience more harmonious manifestations. Conversely, when we become ensnared in the ego-driven narratives of our minds, we confine ourselves within the limitations of those stories. A significant pitfall is the trap of ignorance, which leads to self-imposed restrictions. Those who remain ignorant often accept the constraints imposed by others who are equally ignorant.

For instance, if one believes that $2 + 2 = 4$ is the extent of knowledge, that is all they can impart to others. However, if one seeks deeper understanding—such as questioning the origins of the equation and its broader validity—they transcend these limitations. This journey opens the self to the creator, moving beyond the confines of the ego and the constructs of human thought.

Manifestation originates from a cause, which resides within the human mind, while the effect is observable in the external world. This phenomenon is attributed to energy, as atoms themselves are forms of energy; a concentration of this energy ultimately takes shape as matter.

For instance, when an individual speaks, they are expressing thoughts that were previously unseen or invisible, thereby bringing them into the realm of visibility. What a person harbours internally is what they project outwardly. The listener then has the option to either embrace this energy, allowing it to influence them, or to disregard it. This principle applies equally to beliefs and material objects.

Those who believe in their ability to achieve will manifest that reality, just as those who doubt their capabilities will also bring that belief to fruition. Energy and vibration are constants for all individuals, granting each person the power of choice. Nevertheless, societal conditioning has often led us to *subdue* our inherent gifts, as referenced in some biblical texts.

Power

The concept of power refers to the ability or capacity to guide or sway the actions of others or to shape the course of events. It is essential to understand that power involves influencing the behaviour of individuals.

As self-governing, sovereign beings, we often find ourselves playing roles that may not reflect our true nature. For instance, if an individual were to proclaim loudly in a public space, *"I am a powerful person,"* they might be met with ridicule, with some responding, *"If you are truly powerful, then demonstrate it."*

However, when we delve into the definition of influence, it becomes clear that it encompasses the ability to affect the character, development, or actions of others, as well as the consequential effects of such influence. This is often done in an underhanded way.

Character, in this context, refers to the mentality or role that a person adopts; it signifies a human engaged in action rather than merely existing. Throughout our educational journey, we are often indoctrinated or conditioned from an early age. Rather than being taught about our true selves, we are instructed on how to fit into a predetermined business model.

This conditioning includes notions of obligation, fear, and compliance. Within the confines of the educational system— which can be likened to a prison—we are compelled to adhere to established rules. We absorb societal expectations regarding those who occupy specific character roles, often viewing them through the lens of labels and costumes that dictate whom to admire, trust, or follow. This entire process is orchestrated to manipulate and influence our perceptions.

The individual who asserts their power may not possess genuine influence over you, as they have simply revealed their truth, which you have been conditioned to dismiss. Conversely, those who exert power over you do so primarily because of the early conditioning you have undergone; you have not exercised your own power, thereby allowing them to exercise theirs.

Freedom

Our biggest lesson is to leave nature's creators alone. When one sits in stillness and directs attention to the area between the eyebrows, the surrounding noise begins to fade. In this state, one experiences the essence of existence that transcends time. Attempting to articulate this experience or allowing egoic thoughts to intrude only serves to diminish its purity. Language is inadequate to encapsulate the infinite. The true nature of reality lies beyond the confines of egoic thoughts, words, the physical body, and all belief systems.

My study reveals that we entered a world driven by trade, and our minds have been moulded to serve the interests of those who control business and evil. Rather than recognising our true nature as pure conscious awareness—the ultimate reality—we have come to identify ourselves as physical bodies, influenced by the labels imposed by others. This identification has led to a confinement within the body, creating a metaphorical prison. Although we may sense this confinement and seek freedom, we often inadvertently reinforce it by adhering to the indoctrinations of those who confine us, leading to a form of enslavement.

The labels instilled in us—such as powerful, special, intelligent, and all-knowing—are also forms of indoctrination. They are constructs of a fabricated reality, influenced by the seven deadly sins. We place trust in terms like healthcare, government, and healthy food, among others. However, the manner in which these labels are employed fosters a false sense of security.

I contend that the prayer *"deliver me from evil"* refers to the ego. By relinquishing your own ego, you simultaneously release all egos, fostering inner peace through kindness, compassion, and love for yourself, which naturally extends to others. This awareness allows you to perceive those around you in their own prisons and discomfort.

You do everything to yourself. You let everyone know who you are being. If love comes out of you, you are in a state of love. If jealousy comes out of you, you are in a state of jealousy. If hate comes out of you, you are in a state of hate. These states are all you, and you leak them out to others. This is the law of karma—what you do to others has already been done to you.

To attain true freedom, one must release the indoctrinations rooted in fear, such as the notions of obligation and necessity. By relinquishing doubts, you embody intelligence itself. Without your awareness, the fabricated narratives of the ego cannot persist. These narratives exist solely because of your belief in them. Regardless of the labels you adopt, you validate them through your actions, becoming a mere human-doer, driven by your convictions.

You possess capabilities that extend far beyond this. No individual is superior to you; we are all created equal under the grace of our Creator, made in that divine image to exercise our autonomy. What are you choosing to create? Our Creator has bestowed upon us the resources of this planet for collective enjoyment, not for ownership.

Allow everything to exist as it is and surrender to it, free from the incessant chatter of the ego that seeks to fix, alter, or evade. Perceive the fabricated world of the ego as irrelevant to your true self. Even if you were to spend a month in space, the egoic narrative would remain unchanged.

Consider stepping away from social media and then returning. It resembles a hamster wheel or the repetitive cycle of *Groundhog Day*. Recognising this madness is essential to finding your way out.

Some believe that we must endure the destruction of poisoning our world—meaning our mind, body, and planet—suffering such pain that we are forced to return home. However, I believe that we are already home and have merely been distracted from ourselves by the illusion of evil. Evil does not truly exist unless we fantasise about it. We were informed of this in biblical writings, where Jesus was tempted by Satan.

Do you ever ask why the internal dialogue in your head is so negative and destructive? Your body is not your enemy. Illness arises from the awful experiences—emotional, physical, and psychological—that we hold within it. It is affected by what we consume, our pain, our anger, and our unresolved hurt.

As children, we embody forgiveness, love, and connection. Some call this innocence, yet it is gradually buried beneath the egoic stories imposed upon us as we grow. These stories wipe away our happiness and replace it with fear, obligation, compliance, and the endless weight of *musts* and *shoulds*.

When individuals—both adults and children—seek therapy, it is often to adjust their behaviours to fit societal norms rather than to critically examine those norms. Many fail to recognise the signals conveyed by their bodies, which are often responses to abnormal circumstances.

To evaluate human existence is to evaluate its creator. I am unaware of any person capable of creating another human without utilising the resources provided by that very being. Only wickedness would dare to assess the planet, its climate, and all forms of life with the intent to bring about their destruction or profit. We are made whole; our only job is to realise it.

> *"Not everything that is faced can be changed,*
> *But nothing can be changed until it is faced."*
>
> **James Baldwin.**

Bibliography

- Anderson, J. and Abrahamson, K. (2018). **Your health care may kill you: Medical errors.** [online] Studies in health technology and informatics. Available at: https://pubmed.ncbi.nlm.nih.gov/28186008/.

- ARAB, S. (2024). **MUST SEE ARAB MAN WARNS JAMAICA & AFRICA LEADER** ABOUT THIS IN VIRAL VIDEO. [online] YouTube. Available at: https://youtu.be/Ef__VrfI88k?si=mMOuP5d4f4bziL_Y [Accessed 25 November 2024].

- Black History 365. (n.d.). **How Black Soldiers Helped Britain in First World War.** [online] Available at: https://www.blackhistorymonth.org.uk/article/section/bhm-heroes/how-black-soldiers-helped-britain-in-first-world-war/. [Accessed 14 December 2024].

- Blum, D. (2011). Love at Goon Park: **Harry Harlow and the science of affection.** New York: Basic Books.

- Bowlby, J. (1988). A Secure Base: **Clinical Applications of Attachment Theory.** London: Routledge.

- Chu B, Marwaha K, Sanvictores T, Awosika AO, Ayers D. **Physiology, Stress Reaction.** 2024 May 7. In: StatPearls [Internet]. Treasure Island (FL): StatPearls Publishing; 2024 Jan–. PMID: 31082164.

- Dr Clark David (2024). **The Milk Protein Casein and Bipolar Disorder.** [Online] YouTube. Available at: https://youtu.be/-ZR6zQuJYV0?si=YmBKx0pWGTGuA7RM [Accessed 10 July 2024].

- Claydon, S. (2024). Media Enquiries - **Pesticide Action Network UK.** [online] Pesticide Action Network UK. Available at: https://www.pan-uk.org/media-enquiries/ [Accessed 2 September. 2024].

- Coleman, V. (2020) **Meat Causes Cancer and More Food for Thought.** Independently published.

- **Comparison of Selected Pulse Frequencies from Two Different Electrical Stimulators on Blood Flow in Healthy Subjects.** (2016). Physical Therapy. doi:https://doi.org/10.1093/ptj/68.10.1526.

- Dawkins, R. (2024). **Why Religion is a Scam People are Born Into** | Richard Dawkins. [online] YouTube. Available at: https://youtu.be/yxgphYocj9E?si=2HUVw9B6GGqlgAsf [Accessed 4 Jan. 2025].

- Dennison, R.D. (2005). **Creating an Organizational Culture for Medication Safety.** Nursing Clinics of North America, 40(1), pp.1–23. doi:https://doi.org/10.1016/j.cnur.2004.10.001.

- Emoto, M. (2004). **Healing with Water.** The Journal of Alternative and Complementary Medicine, 10(1), pp.19–21. doi:https://doi.org/10.1089/107555304322848913.

- Dr. Gabor Maté. (2024). **You searched for 'If there's one thing I will never frow accustomed to, is the savages' inability to chastised their children'.** - Dr. Gabor Maté. [online] Available at:
  - https://drgabormate.com/?s=%E2%80%9CIf+there%E2%80%99s+one+thing+I+will+never+frow+accustomed+to%2C+is+the+savages%E2%80%99+inability+to+chastised+their+children%E2%80%9D.+ +[Accessed 10 Dec. 2024].

- Dr. John Campbell (2024). **Batch dependent safety**. [online] YouTube. Available at:
  - https://www.youtube.com/watch?v=nD--4tLmb3w [Accessed 14 November. 2024].

- Fasinu, P.S. and Wilborn, T.W. (2024). Pharmacology education in the medical curriculum: **Challenges and opportunities for improvement**. Pharmacology Research & Perspectives, [online] 12(1).
  - doi:https://doi.org/10.1002/prp2.1178.[Accessed 13 October. 2024].

- Ferber, R. (2006). **Solve Your Child's Sleep Problems**: Revised Edition. Simon and Schuster.

- Fromm Erich, (1955). **The Sane Society 2nd Ed.** (Routledge Classics) Routledge publication.

- Gribble, F.M. and Reimann, F. (2016). **Enteroendocrine Cells: Chemosensors in the Intestinal Epithelium.** Annual Review of Physiology, 78(1), pp.277–299.
    - doi:https://doi.org/10.1146/annurev-physiol-021115-105439.

- Google.com. (2024). **Reporting trends in a regional medication error data-sharing system.** - Google Search. [online] Available at:
    - https://www.google.com/search?q=Reporting+trends+in+a+regional+medication+error+data-sharing+system.&oq=Reporting+trends+in+a+regional+medication+error+data-sharing+system.&gs_lcrp=EgZjaHJvbWUyBggAEEUYOTIGCAEQRRg8MgYIAhBFGDzSAQgyOD AxajBqMagCCLACAQ&sourceid=chrome&ie=UTF-
    - 8 [Accessed 15 October. 2024].

- Harding, D.M. (1984). **Living water.** Victor Schauberger and the secrets of natural energy. Forest Ecology and Management, 7(3), pp.238–239.
    - doi:https://doi.org/10.1016/0378-1127 (84)90073-2.

- Healthydirections.com. (2024). **The Most Dangerous Medications for Your Microbiome.** [online] Available at:

- o https://www.healthydirections.com/articles/digestive-health/most-dangerous-medications-gut-health.
  - o [Accessed 11 October. 2024].
- Healthy Ever After (2024). **The 6 BIGGEST SECRETS They're KEEPING FROM YOU!** Dr. Sebi & Dr. Bobby Price. [online] YouTube. Available at:
  - o https://www.youtube.com/watch?v=9vDdYo2qWWU [Accessed 06 June. 2023].
- Heblich, S., Redding, S. and Voth, H.-J. (2023). **Slavery and the British Industrial Revolution**. [online] CEPR. Available at:
  - o https://cepr.org/voxeu/columns/slavery-and-british-industrial-revolution.
- History.ac.uk. (2007). **Britain, slavery and the trade in enslaved Africans, by Marika Sherwood.** [online] Available at:
  - o https://archives.history.ac.uk/history-in-focus/Slavery/articles/sherwood.html#9t [Accessed 10 August. 2024].
- Hollwich. (1909). **The Influence of Ocular Light Perception on Metabolism In Man and Animals.** Translated by Huner and Hildegard Hannum. Spring Verlag. New York Inc.
- Ibrahim Al-Sawalha, Nebras Jaloudi, Zaben, S., Rawan Hamamreh, Hala Awamleh, S. Al-Abbadi, Abuzaid, L. and

Faisal Abu-Ekteish (2023). **Attitudes of undergraduate medical students toward patients' safety in Jordan:** a multi-center cross-sectional study. BMC Medical Education, [online] 23(1). doi:https://doi.org/10.1186/s12909-023-04672-9.

- Infante, Deliana. (2024). **Beyond Animal Testing: The Rise of Ethical Alternatives in Clinical Research.** AZoLifeSciences. Available at:
  - https://www.azolifesciences.com/article/Beyond-Animal-Testing-The-Rise-of-Ethical-Alternatives-in-Clinical-Research.aspx. [Accessed 7 July. 2024].

- **Intoxicants in Society**. Nih.gov. (2024). Available at:
  - https://openi.nlm.nih.gov/detailedresult?img=PMC4879807_HV-17-42-g005&req=4. [Accessed 7 July. 2024].

- Imperial War Museums (2023). **How Europe Went to War in 1939.** [online] Imperial War Museums. Available at:
  - https://www.iwm.org.uk/history/how-europe-went-to-war-in-1939.

- John Nash Ott (1990). **Health and light** : the effects of natural and artificial light on man and other living things. Columbus, Ohio: Ariel Press.

- Jones, K.A., Cochran, G.L., Hicks, R.J. and Mueller, K.J. (2004). **Translating Research Into Practice:** Voluntary Reporting of Medication Errors in Critical Access Hospitals.

Journal of Rural Health. doi:https://doi.org/10.1111/j.1748-0361.2004.tb00047.x.

- Kellman, R. (2014). **The Microbiome Diet.** Da Capo Lifelong Books.

- Kruse, J. (2013). Epi-paleo Rx : **the prescription for disease reversal and optimal health.** United States: Optimized Life Plc.

- Lucrezia Rovati, Gary, P.J., Edin Cubro, Dong, Y., Oguz Kilickaya, Schulte, P.J., Zhong, X., Malin Wörster, Kelm, D.J., Gajic, O., Niven, A.S. and Lal, A. (2024). **Development and usability testing of a patient digital twin for critical care education:** a mixed methods study. Frontiers in Medicine, 10. doi:https://doi.org/10.3389/fmed.2023.1336897.

- Konrad Lorenz (1970). **Studies in Animal and Human Behaviour.** Cambridge, Mass., Harvard University Press, -71.

- Dr La Mandre (2024). **6 Foods You Should Never Eat.** [Online] YouTube. Available at:
    - https://youtu.be/ZvVLY4LCzHQ?si=t_lwoTC45v1UERBB [Accessed 24 July 2024].

- LuiSpot (2024). **Brave Indian historian brutally shuts the white superiority fallacy.** [online] YouTube. Available at:
    - https://www.youtube.com/watch?v=zNU4Pl-HdnU [Accessed 14 Dec. 2024].

- Macularsociety.org. (2019). **Macular conditions.** [online] Available at:
    - https://www.macularsociety.org/macular-disease/macular-conditions/?gad_source=1&gclid=CjwKCAiAjKu6BhAMEiwAx4UsAlXCncvzBMPyqaabLgRs2Uy5M9Ph_DXlT_qFZ42r3ZPKmr---OxFyxoCn-sQAvD_BwE [Accessed 01 October. 2024].
- Maxwell, J. (2024). Jordan Maxwell: '**The Bible ISN'T What You Think..** Decoding Religious Symbolism' (full explanation). [online] YouTube. Available at:
    - https://youtu.be/UqHSXTxhH24?feature=shared [Accessed 14 October. 2024].
- Neil (2017). **Neil deGrasse Tyson on God.** [online] YouTube. Available at:
    - https://youtu.be/I0nXG02tpDw?si=fTpIAPpkCHTPAgrC [Accessed 14 October. 2024].
- Newman, B. (2023**). The British monarchy's ties to slavery are writ large in the historical archives.** The Guardian. [online] 6 Apr. Available at:
    - https://www.theguardian.com/commentisfree/2023/apr/06/british-monarchy-ties-slavery-historical-archives-slaves. [Accessed 2 August. 2024].

- Not, I. (2023). Hashimoto's Exposed: It's Not Just Your Thyroid, It's a Body-Wide Wake-up Call! [online] YouTube. Available at:
  - https://youtu.be/sNs9vyc4LCo?si=oB-yPtT18kwPeIzw [Accessed 15 Dec. 2024].
- Patrick, K. (2024). How does processed meat cause cancer and how much matters? [online] Cancer Research UK - Cancer News. Available at:
  - https://news.cancerresearchuk.org/2024/08/01/bacon-ham-hot-dogs-salami-how-does-processed-meat-cause-cancer-and-how-much-matters. [Accessed 2 August. 2024].
- Professor Thomas Seyfried (2012**). holds a position as a professor of Biology at Boston College.** Wiley.
- Psichas, A., Sleeth, M.L., Murphy, K.G., Brooks, L., Bewick, G.A., Hanyaloglu, A.C., Ghatei, M.A., Bloom, S.R. and Frost, G. (2014). **The short chain fatty acid propionate stimulates GLP-1 and PYY secretion via free fatty acid receptor 2 in rodents.** International Journal of Obesity, 39(3),
  - Pp.424–429.
  - doi:https://doi.org/10.1038/ijo.2014.153.
- Purdue.edu. (2024). **Search.** [online] Available at:
  - https://docs.lib.purdue.edu/do/search/?q=The%20need%20for%20organizational%20change%20in%20

patient%20safety%20initiatives.&start=0&context=
209723&facet= [Accessed 01 September. 2024].

- Reelblack (2018). **What Color Was Jesus?** (1993) |
  COMPLETE | Donahue w/ Blair Underwood. YouTube.
  Available at:

  o https://www.youtube.com/watch?v=skR7FvtnyLs
    [Accessed 10 Oct. 2023].

- Ramón, S., DeFelipe, J. and Jones, E.G. (1988). **Cajal on
  the Cerebral Cortex.**

- Sitchin. Zecharia, (2019). **The End of Days Armageddon
  and Prophecies of the Return** (Earth Chronicles, Book 7).
  Publisher. Tantor Audio.

- Soul, F. (2021). **The Power of Your Thoughts and The
  Placebo Effect Explained - Bruce Lipton.** YouTube.
  Available at:

  o https://www.youtube.com/watch?v=9LPR-
    Go8JWA [Accessed 15 Jan. 2023].

- Spector, T. (2021). SPOON-FED **: why almost everything
  we've been told about food is wrong.** S.L.: Vintage.

- Steve (2024). **The British Army's Struggle with Systemic
  Racism and Integration.** [online] Wavell Room. Available
  at:

  o https://wavellroom.com/2024/04/11/the-british-
    armys-struggle-with-systemic-racism-and-
    integration/[Accessed 12 December. 2024].

- The (2024). **The Corrupt History of Medicine** | Calley Means. [online] YouTube. Available at:
- https://youtu.be/wT3eVlugPB8?feature=shared [Accessed 7 March. 2024].
- Tomatis, A. (1996). **The ear and language.** Norval, Ontario, Canada: Moulin Publishing.
- Dr. Chris Van Tulleken: **How Ultra-Processed Foods Are Making Us Sick.** [online] YouTube, Available at:
  - https://youtu.be/6SxK9MFmH4c?si=Oo9nfqNxJE_z KH1o [Accessed 7 August 2024].
- United States Holocaust Memorial Museum (2020). **Documenting Numbers of Victims of the Holocaust and Nazi Persecution**. [online] Holocaust Encyclopedia. Available at:
  - https://encyclopedia.ushmm.org/content/en/article/d ocumenting-numbers-of-victims-of-the-holocaust- and-nazi-persecution.
- Vroom, V.H. (1964). **Work and Motivation.** New York : Wiley.
- Waeschle, R.M., Bauer, M. and Schmidt, C.E. (2015). **[Errors in medicine. Causes, impact and improvement measures to improve patient safety].** Der Anaesthetist, [online]
  - 64(9), pp.689–704. doi:https://doi.org/10.1007/s00101-015-0052-4.

- Watson, J.B. (1913). **Psychology as the Behaviourist Views it.** Ardent Media

- We Love Africa (2024**). Russia Opens Centuries-Old Cellars & Reveals Black Biblical Israelites!** [online] YouTube. Available at:
  - https://www.youtube.com/watch?v=9L17tGc5KBk [Accessed 10 December. 2024].

- Dr William Davies (2019) **Wheat Belly. Harper Collins Publication.** London.

- www.ncbi.nlm.nih.gov. (n.d.). Site Map - Site Guide - NCBI. [online] Available at:
  - https://www.ncbi.nlm.nih.gov/guide/sitemap/

- YouTube. (2024). **Dr Sebi Reveals Herbs For Mucus Removal.** [online] Available at:

- https://youtu.be/aJ2yivII_Yo?feature=shared[Accessed 11 February. 2024].

- Youtu.be. (2024). **Watch This Former Big Pharma Lobbyist Expose It All** - YouTube. [online] Available at:
  - https://youtu.be/MQ1PEEu_VZk?feature=shared[Accessed 14 Dec. 2024].

- Zeng, F.-G., Tang, Q., Dimitrijevic, A., Starr, A., Larky, J. and Blevins, N.H. (2011). **Tinnitus suppression by low-rate electric stimulation and its electrophysiological mechanisms.** Hearing Research, 277(1-2), pp.61–66.
  - doi:https://doi.org/10.1016/j.heares.2011.03.010

- Law and, Q. (2024). Questions and Answers. [online] CommonLawConstitution.org. Available at:
  - https://www.commonlawconstitution.org/resources/questions-and-answers. [Accessed 1 October. 2024].
- The Great Seal Act:
  - https://www.legislation.gov.uk/aep/Wi...
- The Treason Act: https://www.legislation.gov.uk/aep/Wi...
- The Act of Wil and Mar:
  - https://www.legislation.gov.uk/aep/Wi...
  - The Coronation Oath 1688:
  - https://www.legislation.gov.uk/aep/Wi...
  - The Bill of Rights 1688:
  - https://www.legislation.gov.uk/aep/Wi...
  - The Act of Settlement 1700:
- https://www.legislation.gov.uk/aep/Wi..
- https://www.legislation.gov.uk/aep/Will3/7-8/3,
- https://www.legislation.gov.uk/ukpga/1967/23
- Wikipedia Contributors (2019). Lord Chancellor. [online] Wikipedia. Available at:
  - https://en.wikipedia.org/wiki/Lord_Chancellor. [Accessed 1 October. 2024].

Constitutional Documents Of Our Right.

- Nolan Principles   Policing principles.
- 2020 Sentencing Act 2010 Equality Act.

- 2006 Police Reform Act 1974 and 1999 Health And Safety Legislation.

- 1886 Promissory Oath Act 1978 Oaths Act.

- 1861 Offences Against the Person Act 1948 Universal Declaration of Humna Rights.

- 1707 Union With England Act 1706 Union with Scotland Act.

- 1700 Act of Settlement 1689 Claim Of Right (Scotland).

- 1688 Bill Of Rights 1688 Act of William and Mary.

- 1567 to 1688 Coronation Oath Act 1628 Petition of Right.

- 1405 and 1423 Confirmation of Liberties 1368 Observance of Due Process of Law.

- 1351 Statute the Fifth 1354 Liberty of the Subject.

- 1361 Justices of the Peace Act   1297 Magna Carta.

- 1215 Magna Carta 1225 Charter of the Forests.

- 893 King Alfred's Dooms 1100 Charter of Liberties.

- Rule of Law Equality Constitutions.

www.ingramcontent.com/pod-product-compliance
Lightning Source LLC
Chambersburg PA
CBHW071714120626

46550CB00001B/234

* 9 7 8 1 9 6 7 1 0 9 4 7 0 *